HEALING *Gourmet*®

Eat to Fight Cancer

THE EDITORS OF HEALING GOURMET WITH

Simin Liu, M.D., Sc.D.,

Kathy McManus, M.S., RD, and John A. Carlino, CEC

McGraw·Hill

New York   Chicago   San Francisco   Lisbon   London   Madrid   Mexico City
Milan   New Delhi   San Juan   Seoul   Singapore   Sydney   Toronto

Library of Congress Cataloging-in-Publication Data

    Healing gourmet, eat to fight cancer / with Simin Liu, Kathy McManus, and John A. Carlino.
        p.   cm.
    Includes bibliograhical references and index.
    ISBN 0-07-145754-2 (alk. paper)
    1. Cancer—Diet therapy—Popular works.   I. Title: Eat to fight cancer.   II. Liu, Simin.   III. McManus, Kathy.   IV. Carlino, John A.   V. Healing gourmet.

RC271.D52 H42   2006
616.99'40654—dc22   2005009864

1 2 3 4 5 6 7 8 9 0 FGR/FGR 0 9 8 7 6 5

ISBN 0-07-145754-2

McGraw-Hill books are available at special quantity discounts to use as premiums and sales promotions, or for use in corporate training programs. For more information, please write to the Director of Special Sales, Professional Publishing, McGraw-Hill, Two Penn Plaza, New York, NY 10121-2298. Or contact your local bookstore.

This book is printed on acid-free paper.

This book is dedicated to cancer patients, survivors, and their families.

Contents

Acknowledgments

THIS BOOK IS brought to you with the assistance and knowledge of medical, culinary, and nutritional experts from across the nation, as well as the diligent work of countless scientists worldwide who help us translate "research to recipes" in our mission to educate on the link between diet and disease. Healing Gourmet would like to thank the following people for their contribution.

A very special thanks to our book editor, Natasha Graf, for her attention to detail and function as a catalyst for many of the concepts presented in this book, and to our project editor, Nancy Hall, for her excellent work in the final editing of the manuscript.

Our medical, nutritional, and culinary editors: Thanks to Dr. Simin Liu for his thorough medical review and guidance; Kathy McManus for her speedy and meticulous work on recipe analysis, meal planning, and nutritional review; and John Carlino for his culinary expertise and recipe testing to ensure that our recipes deliver as much taste as they do health.

Our publisher: Thanks to McGraw-Hill for their ongoing commitment to delivering high-quality information to the public, including their many educational textbooks that spurred the development of this company.

Our affiliations: Thanks to the fine institutions that bring us these editors, including Harvard Medical School, Brigham and Women's Hospital, Dana Farber Cancer Institute, and Florida Culinary Institute.

Our contributors: Thanks to Anne Chiavacci, M.S., M.A., R.D.; Stacy Kennedy, M.P.H., R.D.; Tara Mardigan, M.S., M.P.H., R.D.; and Stephanie Vangsness, M.S., R.D.

Our associates: Thanks to Guy Gelin and our friends and families for their continuing support of the Healing Gourmet project.

Letter from the Editor

CAN SOMETHING AS delicious as Triple Crucifer Soup help to fight cancer? This is just one of the questions we set out to answer nearly five years ago with the creation of our company. Dedicated solely to helping the public make better choices about the foods to eat to prevent disease, Healing Gourmet brings you sound, scientific evidence and practical solutions to help you take control of your health.

Our recipe for health is simple. First, we take a disease-fighting dose of research collected from the National Library of Medicine on your favorite foods, compounds in foods, and their effects on disease. At this very moment, scientists are hard at work analyzing nutrients in foods for their beneficial effects on blood sugar, their cholesterol-lowering capacity, and their cancer-crushing potential. Other researchers are poring over data from population studies to give us clues about why disease rates are lower in other countries where their diets differ greatly from those in the United States. Together, this research in the "new nutritional frontier" acts as the foundation—the first ingredient—in a disease-beating mix.

The next step in our recipe for health is incorporating these scientific findings with culinary finesse to whip up mouthwatering recipes and easy-to-use meal plans that help you make the most of the latest nutritional breakthroughs.

Don't forget to visit us on the Web at healinggourmet.com, and look for us on cable television's Healthy Living Channel. Enjoy these books in good health and *eat your medicine*!

—KELLEY LUNSFORD
    Editor-in-Chief
    Chairman, President, and C.E.O.

Introduction

HEALING GOURMET BEGAN with a mission to educate people on the link between diet and disease. As part of a series, this book is meant to provide useful information on eating to prevent and fight cancer through sound nutritional principles. We bring the "clinic" together with the "kitchen" to help you deliciously make the most of your health through the latest discoveries. Quite simply, Healing Gourmet translates research into recipes, making your kitchen a healing haven.

In this book, we will help you understand the basic principles of cancer and how your diet can help in prevention and aid in recovery. Chapter 1 explains the cancer process and the lifestyle changes you can make to reduce your risk. Chapter 2 focuses on those who have been diagnosed with cancer, what to expect, and how to nurture patients with delicious anticancer foods. Chapters 3 and 4 demystify fats and carbohydrates—showing you how to select the right ones to stave off cancer—and the amazing phytonutrients, antioxidants, and other nutrients that join forces to protect your cells, help your body fight cancer, and boost your immune system. To make sure you're getting the most of these cancer-fighting compounds, Chapters 5 and 6 introduce you to the foods, herbs, and spices that are chock-full of these nutrients.

Of course, we'll help you sleuth out the healthiest products at the grocery store in Chapter 7, help you plan your cancer-fighting meals in Chapter 8, and give you fifty great recipes to get started in Chapter 9. You'll also find recipes to help you cope with possible side effects of treatment. Resources to help with cancer recovery can be found in Chapter 10. Don't forget to visit our website, healinggourmet.com, for the latest research and more cancer-fighting recipes!

IMPORTANT DISCLAIMER: *The information in this book cannot replace the advice of your physician or health-care team. Always consult with your doctor or dietitian before making any changes in your diet.*

About the Contributors

Medical Editor

Simin Liu, M.D., is an associate professor of medicine at Harvard Medical School, Department of Epidemiology, and the director of nutrition research in the Division of Preventive Medicine at Brigham and Women's Hospital. Dr. Liu's work focuses on the effects of nutrition on specific diseases, primarily through large studies, including the Nurses' Health Study, the Women's Health Study, and the Physicians' Health Study.

Nutrition Editor

Kathy McManus, M.S., R.D., is the director of nutrition at Brigham and Women's Hospital, a Harvard teaching affiliate. Ms. McManus is the director of nutrition and behavior modification programs for the program for weight management at the Brigham and is a coinvestigator on a five-year, NIH-funded obesity study, the POUNDS Lost Trial, in collaboration with colleagues at Harvard School of Public Health. In this capacity, she oversees both the inpatient and ambulatory areas of the department. Ms. McManus has extensive experience counseling patients with chronic diseases and has a special interest in weight management.

Culinary Editor

John Carlino, CEC, CCE, FMP, is the chairman of culinary education at the Florida Culinary Institute in West Palm Beach, Florida. With more than fifteen years of experience, Chef Carlino has served as saucier at Spada's Piedmont Lodge in Stratford, Connecticut; the chef saucier at the Century Plaza Hotel in Los Angeles; and the chef/owner of Ives Restaurant Association, which operates three popular Danbury, Connecticut, restaurants (Winslow's, Ciao Café, and Two Steps Downtown Grille). Chef Carlino was recently named Chef of the Year by the American Culinary Federation and was Culinarian of the Year in 1999.

Understanding Cancer and Reducing Your Risk

CANCER IS A GROUP of diseases that begins in our genes. The genes in a healthy body work together, regulating cell division to ensure that each new cell is an exact replica of the parent cell. When cells are damaged and die, they are repaired and replaced in this way. Due to causes that remain largely unknown, mutations in genes lead to cellular chaos—unhealthy cells that grow and divide unchecked to form a mass and thus produce cancer. As the tumor continues to grow, it invades healthy tissue and can spread, or *metastasize*.

A risk factor is anything that increases a person's chance of getting a disease. Different cancers have different risk factors. However, having one risk factor or even several does not necessarily mean that a person will get cancer. Genetic, hormonal, immune, and environmental factors (working either alone or in combination) affect the initiation and promotion of cancer. In this first chapter, we discuss the cellular mutations and DNA damage that lead to cancer, the known risk factors for specific types of cancer, and early warning signs and precancerous conditions to watch for. In understanding your basic risk factors, you will also learn the factors that can improve nutrition and wellness and take steps to reduce your risk of developing cancer.

Genetic Risk Factors for Cancer

Each of us is born with about thirty thousand genes in each cell. Genes are small segments of DNA that control how cells function. A gene can mutate, or become abnormal, and change how the cell grows and divides. Prior to technological advances in modern molecular biology, epidemiologists had found that cancers tend to run in families. In fact, familial aggregation occurs in nearly every form of human cancer. Although some of this aggregation may be due to shared exposure to cancer-causing

TABLE 1.1	**Breast Cancer, Colon Cancer, Prostate Cancer, and Lung Cancer**	
Cancer	**Family History**	**Increase in Cancer Risk**
Breast	Mother diagnosed before age 40	2 times more risk
	Mother diagnosed after age 70	1.5 times more risk
	Sister diagnosed	2 times more risk
Colon	One parent or sibling diagnosed	1.7 times more risk
	Two parents or siblings diagnosed	3 times more risk
Prostate	Father or brother diagnosed	1.5 times more risk
Lung	One parent or sibling diagnosed	2 times more risk

Source: Data from *Harvard Report on Cancer Prevention* 1996.

agents in the environment, the rest is presumably due to inherited mutations in our genes.

In Table 1.1, we illustrate the approximate increase in risk, based on family history, for major types of cancer.

To determine your personal risk for specific cancers, you can also use Harvard's "Your Cancer Risk" interactive risk assessment tool at yourdiseaserisk.harvard.edu.

Hormonal Risk Factors

The most established risk factors for cancer are related to hormone levels, which drive cell division and increase the chances for random DNA copying errors to occur. These errors lead to mutations in genes and the promotion of malignant cell growth.

Estrogen

In looking at some of the hormones involved in the cancer process, estrogen has been shown to be an important growth factor for cells of the breast and ovaries and has been implicated in cancer of reproductive tissues. As a sex steroid, estrogen is believed to drive the proliferation of cells, acting as an important cancer promoter. Factors that increase estrogen exposure (such as alcohol use, obesity after menopause, and postmenopausal hormone use) increase breast cancer risk, while factors that decrease estrogen levels (such as physical activity and breast-feeding) tend to reduce breast cancer risk.

Prolactin

Prolactin is a naturally circulating hormone that is important for lactation and normal breast development. However, it also appears to play a key role in the development and progression of breast cancer. Animal and test-tube models have suggested that a high level of prolactin may act as a cancer promoter and increase tumor growth rates. In the 1999 Nurses' Health Study, researchers found that women with higher prolactin levels were about 40 percent more likely to develop invasive breast cancer than women with lower prolactin levels. It was also found that prolactin levels may be related to the hormone receptor status of breast cancer cells. Hormone receptors are proteins on the surface of some tumor cells. Specific hormones such as estrogen and progesterone can attach to these receptors, causing changes within the cell that stimulate growth. Tumor cells that have hormone receptors are called *hormone-receptor positive*, while those that do not are called *hormone-receptor negative*. In the Nurses' Health Study, prolactin levels were strongly associated with breast cancers that were estrogen-receptor positive but not with those that were estrogen-receptor negative.

Other Hormones

In addition to estrogen, sex steroids include other hormones such as progesterone and androgens like testosterone. Unlike prolactin, these hormones have been evaluated in a number of prospective studies, and almost all of the available data have been pooled for analysis. These pooled data show that the risk of breast cancer increases with increasing blood levels of estrogens and androgens. In the 1999 Nurses' Health Study, for example, researchers examined these associations more closely, looking at tumor subtypes and hormone receptor status. They found that estrogens and androgens increase the risk of the development and spread of breast cancer. These relationships are strongest for tumors that are both estrogen- and progesterone-receptor positive and are most apparent in women who have never taken postmenopausal hormones. Progesterone does not appear to be associated with breast cancer risk in these postmenopausal women, regardless of tumor type or hormone status.

Insulin

Insulin and insulin-like growth factors (IGFs) have been linked to cell development and proliferation and identified as growth factors for cells lining the colon. Chronic excessive exposure to insulin, mainly brought about by obesity, may play a role in the development of colonic carcinoma cells, mammary tissue development, and prostate cancer. Studies have shown that *estradiol* (a type of estrogen) and IGFs may work together in the development of breast cancer.

Investigators from the Harvard School of Public Health, the Karolinska Institute of Stockholm, and the University of Athens studied 150 Greek men to evaluate the role of several hormones that may affect prostate disease. Men with higher levels of IGF-1 had a substantially higher risk of developing prostate cancer.

Reproductive History

A woman's reproductive history, by virtue of the alteration of hormone levels, plays an important role in the development of certain cancers, including breast, ovarian, endometrial, cervical, and colon cancer. In general, reproductive factors include those concerning pregnancy—number of births (parity), age at first birth, and lactation (nursing)—and those that mark a change in a woman's reproductive capacity— including age at menarche and menopause.

Late age at first birth, early age at menarche, late age at menopause, and nulliparity (having no children) are each associated with an increase in breast cancer risk. In addition, nulliparity increases the risk of ovarian cancer and may increase the risk of endometrial cancer.

Immune Factors

Healthy immune systems recognize and destroy foreign cells before they have the chance to multiply out of control and form a tumor. One class of immune cells called *natural killer* (*NK*) cells engulf and destroy abnormal cells before they can cause damage. Certain drugs, specifically those that increase hormones or those that tax the liver, may also initiate or promote cancer. In contrast, many plant compounds known as *phytonutrients* may protect against the development of cancer. Vitamins C and E and selenium bolster immune function.

Dietary Risk Factors

The American Institute for Cancer Research and the World Cancer Research Fund estimate that 30 to 40 percent of all cancers can be prevented with a diet rich in fruits, vegetables, and whole grains, coupled with physical activity and maintenance of appropriate body weight. Much uncertainty remains regarding the optimal dietary composition for cancer prevention; as researchers worldwide continue to study the diet-cancer relationship, we are getting a better understanding every day. Mounting evidence indicates the problems of a typical American or "Western" diet, which is high in processed or red meats and refined carbohydrates and sugar and devoid of many cancer-protective phytonutrients. This Western diet, in conjunction with a lack of physical activity, contributes to weight gain, obesity, and hormonal changes that can promote hormone-dependent cancers.

Red Flags: What to Watch For

Being aware of your age, heredity, and lifestyle risk factors is only one part of improving your preventive effort in reducing your risk.

It is equally important that you become aware of the signs that may indicate you have a specific type of cancer. The following sections will provide you with some warning signs to watch for that can be a sign of breast cancer, colorectal cancer, or prostate cancer. Remember, early detection may be the key to survival.

Detecting Breast Cancer: Finding a Lump

You should see your health-care provider if you discover any changes in a breast, changes that persist after your menstrual cycle, or other changes that you are concerned about. Conditions that should be checked by a doctor include the following:

- An area that is distinctly different from any other area on either breast
- A lump or thickening in or near the breast or under the arm that persists throughout your menstrual cycle
- A change in the size, shape, or contour of the breast
- A mass or lump that may feel as small as a pea
- A marblelike area under the skin
- A change in the feel or appearance of the skin on the breast or nipple (dimpled, puckered, scaly, or inflamed)
- Bloody or clear fluid discharge from the nipple
- Redness of the skin on the breast or nipple

Although there are disagreements among experts, the following guidelines for examinations are generally recommended by several national authorities, including the American Cancer Society (cancer.org).

- Monthly breast **self-examinations** should begin at age twenty.
- Breast examinations by a **health-care provider** should be done every three years starting at age twenty; annual clinical breast exams start at age forty.

❖ A **baseline mammogram** should be done at age thirty-five.

❖ **Annual screening mammography** should start at age forty. Women in high-risk categories may want to consider starting screening at age thirty.

Colorectal Cancer: Changes in Bowels

One of the early symptoms of colon cancer may be bleeding. Often, tumors bleed only a little, off and on, and evidence of the blood is found only during chemical testing of the stool. When tumors have grown larger, other symptoms may develop, including the following:

❖ **A change in bowel habits.** Constipation, diarrhea, narrow stools, and bowel incontinence, although usually symptoms of other less serious problems, can possibly be signs of colorectal cancer.

❖ **Blood on or in the stool.** By far the most alarming of all associated symptoms, blood on or in the stool can be an indication of colorectal cancer. However, it does not necessarily mean cancer, as there are numerous other problems that can cause bleeding in the digestive tract, including hemorrhoids, ulcers, ulcerative colitis, and Crohn's disease. In addition, iron and some foods, such as beets, can give the stool a black or red appearance, which can be mistaken for blood. However, if you notice blood in your stool, see your doctor to rule out a serious condition and to ensure proper treatment.

❖ **Unexplained anemia.** Anemia is a shortage of the red blood cells that carry oxygen throughout the body. If you are anemic, you will most likely feel tired and sluggish, so much so that rest does not make you feel better.

❖ **Other symptoms.** Other symptoms to watch for include unusual stomach or gas pain, unexplained weight loss, fatigue, and vomiting.

Unfortunately, colorectal cancer may strike without symptoms. For this reason, it is very important to have regular examinations, called *colorectal screenings*, to detect early problems. Those with average risk should begin prevention examinations at age fifty under the following screening guidelines to detect early-stage lesions and polyps:

❖ **Fecal occult blood test.** This test examines the stool for blood not easily noticed by the naked eye. For those at average risk of colorectal cancer, this test should be given every year starting at age fifty along with a flexible sigmoidoscopy every five years. *Flexible sigmoidoscopy* is a routine outpatient procedure in which a physician uses a sigmoidoscope (a long, flexible instrument about half an inch in diameter) to view the lining of the rectum and the lower third of the large intestine (called the sigmoid and descending colon).

❖ **Air contrast barium enema.** This test is an X-ray examination of the entire colon and rectum in which barium and air are introduced gradually into the colon by a rectal tube to improve visualization. Doctors typically recommend this test in combination with a flexible sigmoidoscopy every five to ten years, starting at age fifty.

❖ **Colonoscopy.** This is an outpatient procedure in which the rectum and the inside of the entire colon are examined. During a colonoscopy, a doctor uses a long, flexible instrument about half an inch in diameter to view the lining of the colon. This test is recommended every ten years (starting at age fifty) unless a polyp is found, at which point doctors recommend a colonoscopy every five years.

Prostate Disease: Urine Troubles

There are three different types of prostate disease: benign prostatic hyperplasia, prostatitis, and prostate cancer. Although these diseases have different causes, they have similar symptoms. For this reason, it's important to be checked for prostate cancer as part of your yearly physical examination and to see a urologist (a doctor who specializes in diseases of the urinary tract and the male reproductive system). We will review the warning signs of each type of prostate disease.

Warning Signs of Benign Prostatic Hyperplasia. Commonly called BPH, *benign prostatic hyperplasia* is a noncancerous enlargement of the prostate gland that affects approximately half of all men at some point before the age of fifty and 80 percent of men after age sixty. The symptoms of BPH include the following:

* Difficulty urinating
* An urge to urinate even when the bladder is empty
* Frequent urination, especially at night
* A weak or intermittent stream of urine and a sense of incomplete emptying after urinating

Warning Signs of Prostatitis. *Prostatitis* is an inflammation of the prostate that can be caused by bacterial infection in men of all ages. The following symptoms may indicate prostatitis:

* Difficulty urinating
* Frequent urination, especially at night
* Pain or burning during urination
* Chills and fever with urinating problems

Warning Signs of Prostate Cancer. In its early stages, prostate cancer may not cause any symptoms. However, as it progresses, symptoms may include the following:

* A need to urinate frequently, especially at night
* Difficulty starting urination

❖ An inability to urinate
❖ A weak or interrupted flow of urine (dribbling)
❖ Painful or burning urination
❖ Painful ejaculation
❖ Blood in urine or semen
❖ Frequent pain or stiffness in the back, hips, or upper thighs

To help detect prostate cancer early, the American Urological Association and the American Cancer Society recommend annual screening for men ages fifty to seventy. They further recommend that men who are at high risk—such as African American men and those with a family history of prostate cancer— begin screening at about age forty. There are two main tests to screen for prostate cancer:

❖ **Prostate-specific antigen (PSA) screening.** A PSA exam is a blood test that measures the amount of PSA (produced by the prostate) in the bloodstream.

❖ **Digital rectal exam (DRE).** The DRE is used to detect prostate cancer in its early stages, when treatment is most successful. Because the prostate is an internal organ lying in front of the rectum, it can be felt with a lubricated, gloved finger inserted into the rectum.

Empowering Wellness

By understanding the lifestyle factors associated with the development of cancer, we can take control of our health to work toward nutritional healing and reduce our risk for cancer occurrence or recurrence. In this next section, we explore how our culinary choices, body weight, exercise, and other lifestyle decisions (such as smoking or consuming alcohol) affect our treatment and risk.

Culinary Choices and Cancer

Over the past few decades, scientists have taken advantage of technological advances to discover new compounds in foods that can promote health and protect us from disease. These compounds, called phytonutrients (plant chemicals), exhibit an array of health-promoting properties—from antioxidant activity to balancing blood sugar.

It should come as no surprise that the foods that help us in recovery and offer us protection come from plants, the very fare our Paleolithic ancestors subsisted on. In fact, our *genome*, or collection of genes, has changed little since the beginning of agriculture. Because of this, we are adapted to eat the same foods as our hunter-gatherer ancestors. In addition, as we deviate from a diet based on plant foods and choose readily accessible high-fat, low-fiber "fast" foods, red and processed meats, sweets and desserts, and refined foods, our risk increases not only for cancer, but also for obesity, inflammation, insulin resistance, and many other chronic conditions known as "diseases of Westernization." For example, the 2003 Nurses' Health Study showed that this Western diet pattern was associated with a 46 percent increase in colon cancer risk in women. Throughout this book, we explain how these foods individually and collectively affect our hormones, immune function, and biochemistry. We discuss the benefits of antioxidants and phytonutrients (Chapter 4) and provide foods (Chapter 5), meal plans (Chapter 8), and recipes (Chapter 9) that help you incorporate more of these important nutrients to your diet.

Weight Matters: A Fat Risk

Obesity has reached epidemic proportions in the United States. Sixty-four percent of the adult population is overweight or obese and 1 in 50 is severely obese. Scientists believe that obesity and being overweight account for up to 14 percent of all cancer deaths in nonsmoking men and up to 20 percent of those in nonsmoking women, and that more than ninety thousand cancer deaths per year could be avoided by maintaining proper weight. We can achieve a healthy weight by choosing fruits, vegetables, legumes, and whole (not refined) grains as our dietary staples; limiting portions; and avoiding energy-dense, nutrient-depleted foods. In Chapter 9, you'll find recipes that incorporate lots of vegetables and fruits to help you on the road to recovery and prevention.

In addition to eating the wrong things, "portion distortion" is everywhere. What most Americans don't realize is that super-sized meals lead to super-sized health problems. The portion size at most fast-food restaurants has increased, and studies show that people will eat more when presented with a bigger portion. Worse yet, Americans underestimate the number of calories they consume by 25 to 50 percent. Fifty excess calories a day over a ten-year period will increase your weight by fifty pounds! Conversely, cutting 100 calories a day means you will drop seven pounds in a year.

Food isn't the only culprit, however. Soda guzzling can tack on calories and pounds as well. How can refined foods lead to overeating? Studies have shown that the outer layers of grain, called bran and germ layers, contain both fiber and important nutrients. Refining a grain removes those important layers, causing the starchy inside, or endosperm, to come into direct contact with our mucous membranes. The refined grain is digested more quickly, sending sugar into the bloodstream, which in turn causes hormonal and metabolic changes that promote hunger. We discuss refined grains, the glycemic index, and their implications for health further in Chapter 3.

What is the link between being overweight or obese and developing cancer? Weight gain as an adult is an important determinant of both breast and colon cancers, and significant positive associations have been found between obesity and higher death rates for cancers of the esophagus, colon and rectum, liver, gallbladder, pancreas, kidney, stomach (in men), prostate, breast, cervix, uterus, and ovaries. The European Prospective Investigation into Cancer and Nutrition (EPIC) found that body mass index (BMI) and hip ratio were positively associated with breast cancer risk, and women with a BMI greater that 30 (obese) increased their risk for breast cancer by 31 percent compared to women with a BMI less than 25. Another study conducted at Boston University found that a BMI greater than 30 was associated with a 50 percent increased risk of colon cancer among middle-aged adults (thirty to fifty-four years) and a 2.4-fold increased risk in older adults (fifty-five to seventy-nine years). This study also found that having a waist circumference greater than or equal to 39 inches for women and 40 inches for men increased colon cancer risk twofold. Researchers believe that an increased exposure to estrogen, as well as insulin and IGFs, in overweight or obese people promote cancer occurrence and recurrence.

Exercise: Rx for Cellular Health

Exercise has been found to afford protection against certain cancers, possibly through weight control, along with a reduction in insulin resistance and exposure to estrogen. The evidence is most consistent for colon cancer, which is reduced by 40 to 50 percent among the most active individuals, compared with those who are the least active. Although the evidence is less consistent, studies suggest a 25 to 30 percent reduction in breast cancer among the most active women.

The U.S. surgeon general, in a report titled "Physical Activity and Health," calls on Americans to use exercise as a "passport to health" and notes the extensive health benefits of regular physical activity, including the following:

* Enhances the overall quality and length of life
* Protects against cardiovascular disease
* Reduces the risk of cancers, specifically of the breast and colon
* Reduces the risk of adult-onset (type 2) diabetes
* Keeps bones strong and helps prevent osteoporosis
* Helps to maintain muscle strength, as well as joint structure and function
* Reduces the risk of falls in the elderly
* Controls weight and positively affects body fat distribution
* Relieves depression and anxiety and improves mood

By reducing hormone levels, keeping our insulin receptors sensitive and functioning properly to metabolize glucose (blood sugar), producing endorphins ("feel-good" neurotransmitters that reduce stress), and reducing body fat to achieve a healthy weight, exercise is an important ingredient in the recipe for health.

Nix the Cancer Sticks: Butt Out

It's no surprise that smoking causes lung cancer, but the story doesn't end there. In fact, smoking is a major risk factor for many other forms of cancer, as the by-products of smoking must travel though the body, beginning at the lips and mouth, traversing air passageways, circulating through the bloodstream, undergoing processing by the liver, and finally being eliminated via the colon (or bladder).

Smoking produces *polycyclic aromatic hydrocarbons* (*PAHs*) in the body. These dangerous compounds, in conjunction with many others, are known to increase the risk for cancers of the lung, oropharynx, stomach, pancreas, kidney, cervix, bladder, pelvis, liver, and colon. It has been estimated that one-third of all cancer deaths in Western countries are caused by smoking and that one-half of all smokers will die from tobacco-related causes.

Alcohol: Proceed with Caution

Excessive consumption of alcohol is the third leading cause of preventable deaths in the United States and is associated with multiple adverse health consequences, including liver cirrhosis, various cancers, unintentional injuries, and violence. Experts urge us to imbibe moderately if we choose to drink. However, the definition of "moderate" has been debated. In some studies, the term *moderate drinking* refers to less than one drink per day, while in others it means three to four drinks per day. Exactly what constitutes "a drink" is also questionable. In fact, even among alcohol researchers, there's no universally accepted standard drink definition. In the United States, one drink is usually considered to be 12 ounces of beer, 5 ounces of wine, or 1½ ounces of spirits (hard liquor such as gin or whiskey). Each delivers approximately 12 to 14 grams of alcohol.

In support of alcohol, more than a hundred prospective studies show an inverse association between moderate drinking and risk of heart attack, ischemic (clot-caused) stroke, peripheral vascular disease, sudden cardiac death, and death from all cardiovascular causes. Not only does moderate alcohol consumption increase high-density lipoprotein (HDL, or "good cholesterol"), but it also reduces the stickiness of platelets that can form a dangerous clot. This effect has been most associated with red wine, due in part to phytonutrients called *polyphenolics*.

The bad news is that alcohol increases certain hormones in the body and decreases vitamins essential to the proper growth and development of cells, which can encourage the development of cancer. Oral cancers are six times more common in alcohol users than in those who abstain, and about 75 to 80 percent of all oral cancer patients consume alcohol regularly. The primary cause of liver cancer is alcohol. By altering the liver's ability to metabolize some cancer-causing agents into harmless compounds or by impairing its ability to deactivate existing carcinogens, alcohol's effects may influence not only liver cancer, but other cancers as well. An additional risk factor for women consuming alcohol is the use of hormone replacement therapy (HRT). Researchers postulate that women using postmenopausal hormones who have one alcoholic beverage daily increase their risk for breast cancer from 4 to 8 percent. If you do choose to drink alcohol, it's important to get at least 400 micrograms of folate each day, as researchers have found that folate helps to reduce the risk of breast cancer in women who drink alcohol. Learn more about how folate protects against cancer in Chapter 4.

Because each of us has unique personal and family histories, alcohol offers each person a different spectrum of benefits and risks. If you don't drink, there's no need to start. You can achieve similar benefits with exercise or healthier eating. If you already drink alcohol or plan to begin, limit it to no more than two drinks a day for men or one drink a day for women. And make sure you get plenty of folate—at least 400 micrograms a day.

Now that we have explored the risk factors associated with cancer, we'll discuss the critical role of diet, both in your diagnosis and in prevention.

Diet and Your Diagnosis

WHEN YOU ARE diagnosed with cancer, so many things go through your mind. What are my treatment options? Will the treatment work? Will my cancer return? Having a positive attitude and empowering yourself with information greatly increases your chances of beating cancer. So does nourishing your body at this critical time to speed your recovery.

Research shows that good food is good medicine, and 20 to 40 percent of cancer deaths may result from nutrition-related issues rather than the disease itself. Eating well during your treatment can help you feel better, improve energy, maintain a proper body weight, tolerate treatment-related side effects, reduce your risk of infection, and hasten healing. While the recommendations for people who have cancer can vary during different stages of treatment and specific nutritional deficiencies, they usually include the same principles as those for preventing cancer:

* Eat five or more servings of fruits and vegetables every day. (See Chapter 4 for the cancer-fighting nutrients in plants and how they work.)
* Choose whole grains as opposed to refined grains. (See Chapter 3 to learn about the difference and how it affects the cancer process.)

* Limit consumption of red meats, especially those high in fat and those that are processed. (See Chapter 3.)
* Choose foods that help you maintain a healthy weight. (We list many beneficial foods in Chapter 5 and provide healthy tips and suggestions for recipes in Chapter 9.)
* Stay well-hydrated.

The Benefits of Nutritional Counseling

While this book provides useful information on the beneficial role of diet in cancer prevention and healing, nutritional counseling offers personalized health benefits for cancer patients both during treatment and in the prevention of recurrence. A recent study conducted at the University of California, San Diego, found that individualized dietary counseling can promote a healthy weight and the inclusion of proper nutrients in the diet; reduce side effects, including anorexia and diarrhea; and improve quality of life. It can also foster the continuation of care through the entire cancer process from diagnosis to remission in the goal to prevent cancer recurrence or the development of other diseases (also known as comorbidities).

Similarly, the Women's Healthy Eating and Living (WHEL) Study found that dietary counseling may play a beneficial role in reducing the recurrence of breast cancer. In this study, telephone counseling was used as a tool to encourage participants who had survived breast cancer to consume a diet emphasizing fruits and vegetables rich in carotenoids and other phytonutrients. At the end of the study, the participants receiving the telephone counseling had increased their consumption of phytonutrient-rich foods by 82 percent. The researchers then analyzed the levels of these compounds in participants' blood and found a 223 percent increase in alpha-carotene, an 87 percent increase in beta-carotene, a 27 percent increase in lutein, and a 17 percent increase in lycopene. Those who did not receive the intervention did not have a significant change in the levels of cancer-fighting phytonutrients in their blood. You can learn about these beneficial compounds and how they can reduce your risk and aid in treatment in Chapter 4.

Nutrition During Treatment

In this section, we'll discuss some strategies to maintain proper nutrition during specific cancer treatments and guide you toward understanding how foods play a role in the cancer process.

Nutrition After Surgery

The body needs additional protein and extra calories to help repair at this time. Most health-care providers recommend beginning with clear liquids:

* Broth, vegetable or chicken
* Tea
* Sports drinks or diluted sports drink
* Strained citrus juices and other juices
* Water

The next step is easy-to-digest foods:

* Instant oatmeal or other hot cereals
* Canned fruits and vegetables
* Lean, moist meats
* Yogurt and milk, Lactaid milk, or soy milk
* Smoothies and milk shakes (You can find many recipes for smoothies in Chapter 9.)

The third step is to ease back into your regular diet. Try to eat minimeals more often, and avoid heavy foods or large meals at this time.

You may experience mouth soreness, difficulty swallowing or chewing, heartburn, indigestion, and diarrhea after surgery, which makes soups and smoothies a perfect option to get your nutrition in liquid form.

Nutrition During Chemotherapy

Chemotherapeutic drugs kill not only cancer cells, but also living tissue and immune cells. Because of this, it is especially important to pay close attention to your diet to ensure you're giving your body the fuel it needs to repair cells, boost your immune system, and prevent complications. Loss of appetite is probably the number-one complaint among cancer patients undergoing chemotherapy. Changes in smell and taste, mouth sores, nausea, vomiting, changes in bowel habits, fatigue, weight loss or gain, and low white blood cell count are also prevalent.

Eating a light meal or snack prior to treatment may help reduce some of the side effects. Small, frequent meals are a good way to keep your energy up and ensure you're getting the nutrition you need. They also make eating less daunting at a time when your appetite is lacking or you are nauseated.

Nutrition During Radiation Therapy

The type of side effects you experience during this treatment depends on the area of radiation, the size of the area being irradiated, and the number of treatments. Much like other treatments, side effects include difficulty swallowing, sore throat, nausea, vomiting, and diarrhea.

Preparing foods in advance—soups, puddings, cereals, and other easy-to-tolerate choices—in small portions and freezing them will make cooking easier when you're not feeling well. You may want to purchase canned vegetable or chicken broth, freeze it in ice trays, and store the cubes in a freezer bag. When you're ready, put a couple in a bowl and reheat. Eating small meals also helps to ease digestion.

Your doctor or health care provider may have recommended extra calories and protein at this time. Those calories and protein should come from lean meats, legumes, good-quality fats (like nut butters and olive oil), and whole grains. Be careful not to choose high-calorie foods that are only sugar.

Coping with Side Effects

During the treatment process there are numerous additional side effects that you may be dealing with. Here are some practical tips for dealing with the side effects of the treatments we described earlier, as well as some recipe suggestions to help get you through your treatment.

Anorexia

Anorexia (lack of appetite) is one of the most common problems for cancer patients. Here are some tips for getting the nutrients you need when you don't want to eat:

* Eat small, high-protein, high-calorie meals every one to two hours instead of three larger meals.
* Get help with preparing meals.
* Add extra calories and protein (such as oils, skim milk powder, and honey) to food.
* Drink liquid supplements (special drinks containing nutrients), soups, milk, juices, shakes, and smoothies when eating solid food is a problem.

❖ Eat snacks that contain plenty of calories and protein.
❖ Prepare and store small portions of favorite foods so they are ready to eat when you're hungry.
❖ Eat breakfasts that contain one-third of the calories and protein needed for the day. A dietitian can help you figure out what your specific calorie and protein needs are.
❖ Eat foods that smell good to you.
❖ Try new foods. Be creative with desserts. Experiment with recipes, flavorings, spices, and types and consistencies of food. Your food likes and dislikes may change from day to day.

 Kitchen Prescription

Feeling Souper! Our Double Veggie Chicken Soup recipe is a great high-protein option and an old-fashioned feel-good remedy. Or turn on the blender—our Super Protein Smoothie delivers 23 grams of protein to help rebuild your cells.

Taste Changes

Changes in how foods taste may be caused by cancer treatment, dental problems, or medicines. Drinking plenty of fluids, changing the types of foods you eat, and adding spices or flavorings to food may help. Check out Chapter 6 for more information on healing herbs and spices. In addition, try the following suggestions:

❖ Rinse your mouth with water before eating.
❖ Try citrus fruits (oranges, tangerines, lemons, grapefruit) unless you have mouth sores.
❖ Eat small meals and healthy snacks several times a day. (In our meal plans in Chapter 8, we include three meals and three snacks a day.)
❖ Eat meals when you're hungry rather than at set mealtimes.

❖ Use plastic utensils if foods taste metallic.

❖ Try your favorite foods.

❖ Eat with family and friends.

❖ Have others prepare the meal.

❖ Try new foods when you feel good.

❖ Substitute poultry, fish, eggs, and cheese for red meat.

❖ Use nonmeat, high-protein recipes.

❖ Use sugar-free lemon drops, gum, or mints if there is a metallic or bitter taste in your mouth.

❖ Add spices and sauces to foods.

 Kitchen Prescription

Get Energized! Our Energizing Smoothie includes grapefruit and oranges. Unless you are dealing with mouth sores or irritations, these fruits in a smooth sherbet base can help you cope with taste changes.

Dry Mouth

Dry mouth is often caused by radiation therapy to the head and neck. Certain medicines may also be to blame. The main treatment for dry mouth is drinking plenty of liquids, about half an ounce per pound of body weight per day. For example, a 150-pound person would drink 75 fluid ounces daily. Other suggestions to manage dry mouth include the following:

❖ Eat moist foods with smooth textures.

❖ Suck on hard candy or chew gum.

❖ Eat frozen desserts (such as frozen grapes and ice pops) or ice chips.

❖ Clean your teeth (including dentures) and rinse your mouth at least four times per day (after each meal and before bedtime).

✤ Keep water handy at all times to moisten your mouth.
✤ Avoid liquids and foods that contain a lot of sugar.
✤ Avoid mouth rinses containing alcohol.
✤ Drink fruit nectar instead of juice.
✤ Use a straw to drink liquids.

Mouth Sores and Infections

Mouth sores can result from chemotherapy and radiation therapy. Choosing certain foods and taking good care of your mouth, with guidance from your treatment team, will make eating easier. Try the following foods:

✤ Soft fruits—including bananas, applesauce, and watermelon
✤ Peach, pear, and apricot nectars
✤ Cottage cheese
✤ Mashed potatoes
✤ Custards or puddings
✤ Smoothies or milk shakes
✤ Scrambled eggs
✤ Oatmeal or other cooked cereals
✤ Vegetables (such as potatoes, peas, and carrots) and meats processed in the blender until smooth

Avoiding the following foods should also help ease the pain of this side effect:

✤ Rough, coarse, or dry foods, including raw vegetables, granola, toast, and crackers
✤ Foods that are spicy or salty
✤ Acidic foods, such as vinegar, pickles, and olives
✤ Citrus fruit or juices, including oranges, grapefruit, and tangerines

In addition, try these tips and techniques when cooking:

* ❖ Cook foods until soft and tender.
* ❖ Cut foods into small pieces.
* ❖ Use a straw to drink liquids.
* ❖ Eat foods cold or at room temperature. Hot and warm foods can irritate a tender mouth.
* ❖ Clean your teeth (including dentures) and rinse your mouth at least four times per day (after each meal and before bedtime). Your doctor can help you determine the best plan for keeping your mouth clean.
* ❖ Add gravy, broth, or sauces to food.
* ❖ Drink high-calorie, high-protein drinks in addition to your meals.
* ❖ Numb your mouth with ice chips.

Nausea

Nausea caused by treatments can limit the nutrients your body needs to battle cancer. Try these suggestions to ease your nausea and fight disease:

* ❖ Eat a small meal or snack before treatments.
* ❖ Avoid foods that are likely to trigger nausea. For some patients, this includes spicy foods, greasy foods, and foods that have strong odors.
* ❖ Eat small meals several times a day.
* ❖ Slowly sip fluids throughout the day.
* ❖ Eat dry foods such as crackers, breadsticks, or toast throughout the day.
* ❖ Sit up or lie with your upper body raised for one hour after eating.
* ❖ Eat bland, soft, easy-to-digest foods rather than heavy meals.

❖ Avoid eating in a room that has cooking odors or that is overly warm. Keep your living space at a comfortable temperature and ventilated with plenty of fresh air.

❖ Rinse out your mouth before and after eating.

❖ Suck on hard candies such as peppermints or lemon drops if your mouth has a bad taste.

❖ Sip a cup of warm ginger tea, or try adding a few slices of fresh gingerroot to warm water or a favorite soothing herbal tea.

 Kitchen Prescription

Ease Your Queasiness! Try our Tummy-Soothing Smoothie with ginger and apricots to settle your stomach and deliver a healthy dose of nutrients.

Diarrhea

Diarrhea may be caused by cancer treatments, surgery on the stomach or intestines, or by emotional stress. Long-term diarrhea may lead to dehydration (lack of water in the body) and/or low levels of salt and potassium—important minerals needed by the body. These suggestions may help to ease symptoms:

❖ Try broth, soups, sports drinks, bananas, and canned fruits to help replace salt and potassium lost by diarrhea.

❖ Avoid greasy foods, hot or cold liquids, and caffeine.

❖ Avoid high-fiber foods—especially dried beans and cruciferous vegetables (such as broccoli, cauliflower, and cabbage).

❖ Drink plenty of fluids throughout the day. Room temperature liquids may cause fewer problems than hot or cold liquids.

❖ Limit milk to two cups or eliminate milk and milk products until the source of the problem is found.

❖ Limit gas-forming foods and beverages such as peas, lentils, cruciferous vegetables, chewing gum, and soda.

❖ Limit sugar-free candies or gum made with sugar alcohols such as mannitol, sorbitol, xylitol, lactitol, isomalt, malitol, and hydrogenated starch hydrolysates (HSH).

❖ Drink at least one cup of liquid shortly after each loose bowel movement.

 Kitchen Prescription

Grab a Straw! Try our Hydrating Smoothie to ease diarrhea and provide electrolytes to prevent dehydration.

Low White Blood Cell Count

Cancer patients may have a low white blood cell count for a variety of reasons—some of which include radiation therapy, chemotherapy, or the cancer itself—which increases the risk of infection. Help reduce this risk with the following tips:

❖ Check the dates on food and do not buy or use the food if it is out of date.

❖ Do not buy or use food in cans that are swollen, dented, or damaged.

❖ Thaw foods in the refrigerator or microwave. Never thaw foods at room temperature. Cook foods immediately after thawing.

❖ Refrigerate all leftovers within two hours of cooking and eat them within twenty-four hours.

❖ Keep hot foods hot and cold foods cold.

❖ Avoid old, moldy, or damaged fruits and vegetables.

✤ Avoid unpackaged tofu sold in open bins or containers.
✤ Cook all meat, poultry, and fish thoroughly. Avoid raw eggs and raw fish.
✤ Buy foods packed as single servings to avoid leftovers.
✤ Avoid salad bars or buffets.
✤ Avoid large indoor public gatherings or wear a mask.
✤ Wash your hands often to prevent the spread of bacteria.

Dehydration

The body needs plenty of water to replace the fluids lost every day. Long-term diarrhea, nausea and vomiting, and pain may prevent you from drinking and eating enough to get the water your body needs. One of the first signs of dehydration is extreme tiredness. The following suggestions may help you prevent dehydration:

✤ Check with your doctor or dietitian about your specific fluid requirements. Fluids include water, juice, milk, or foods that contain a large amount of liquid—such as puddings, ice cream, ice pops, flavored ices, and gelatins.
✤ Take a water bottle whenever you leave home. Drink even if you're not thirsty, as thirst is not a good sign of fluid needs.
✤ Limit drinks that contain caffeine, such as sodas, coffee, and caffeinated tea (both hot and cold).
✤ Drink most liquids after and/or between meals.

Constipation

Constipation is defined as fewer than three bowel movements per week. It is a very common problem for cancer patients and may result from lack of water or fiber in the diet, lack of physical activity, anticancer treatment such as chemotherapy, and medications.

Preventing constipation is a part of cancer care; the following suggestions may help:

❖ **Eat more fiber-containing foods on a regular basis.** The recommended fiber intake is 25 to 35 grams per day. Increase fiber gradually and drink plenty of fluids at the same time to keep the fiber moving through your intestines.

❖ **Drink eight to ten cups of fluid each day.** Water, prune juice, warm juices, lemonade, and teas without caffeine can be very helpful.

❖ **Take walks and exercise regularly.** Proper footwear is important.

If constipation does occur, the following suggestions for diet, exercise, and medication may help correct it:

❖ **Continue to eat high-fiber foods and drink plenty of fluids.** Try adding wheat bran to your diet; begin with 2 heaping tablespoons each day for three days and then increase by 1 tablespoon each day until constipation is relieved. However, do not exceed 6 tablespoons per day.

❖ **Maintain physical activity.**

❖ **Include over-the-counter constipation treatments, if necessary.** This refers to bulk-forming products (such as Benefiber, Citrucel, Metamucil, Fiberall, FiberCon, and Fiber-Lax), stimulants (such as Dulcolax tablets or suppositories and Senokot), stool softeners (such as Colace, Surfak, and Dialose), and osmotics (such as milk of magnesia). Cottonseed and aerosol enemas can also help relieve the problem. Lubricants such as mineral oil are not recommended because they may prevent the body's absorption of important nutrients. Talk with your doctor about what might work for you.

Kitchen Prescription

Running Smoothly! Try our Full of Fiber Smoothie with dates, bananas, and bran to get things running smoothly.

We hope these nutritional and other suggestions will help you deal with some of the side effects as you go through the difficult cancer treatment process. The next few chapters zero in on the foods that will continue to help you with traditional cancer treatments and aid in the prevention of occurrence and recurrence.

Fats, Carbs, and Cancer

MIXED MESSAGES ON fats and carbohydrates have led many Americans to make undesirable food choices. First we hear that fat is bad and carbohydrates (or carbs) are good. Then we are fed the notion that severely limiting carbs—and all the wonderfully nutritious foods in which they are found—will help us lose weight, and a healthy weight is a key factor in preventing diseases, including cancer. These efforts, however, have proven unsuccessful, as an astounding 60 percent of Americans are still overweight or obese. Certain fats and carbohydrates play a key role in health promotion.

A new system for classifying carbs, called the glycemic index, gives us greater insight into the "all carbs are bad" myth and helps us separate the wheat from the chaff (no pun intended). By measuring how fast and how far blood sugar rises after consuming a carb-rich food, we better understand that food's impact on hormones and other key factors that influence disease risk.

Although such a system does not exist for fats, numerous studies have proven the villains and victors of the fat world. Some fats increase cholesterol and make platelets sticky—increasing the risk for a heart attack or stroke—while others allow the arteries to open up and increase levels of "good cholesterol." Although the types of fat we choose are important for overall health, the link between dietary fat and cancer is a weaker case.

When you eliminate good carbs and good fats, you also forgo the critical nutrients that help fight cancer. Do you skip the olive oil, nuts, and avocados because you're afraid of fat? You're missing out on minerals like magnesium, as well as cancer-fighting phytonutrients such as beta-sitosterol and phenols, plus antioxidants such as glutathione. (We discuss phytonutrients and antioxidants further in Chapter 4.) Are you under the impression that all carbs are bad? There goes the fiber that works to support a healthy immune system.

Healing Gourmet makes it easy for you to follow the principles discovered by modern science in preventing and alleviating cancer. In this chapter, we will point out the good guys and bad guys of the fat and carb world and how they relate to cancer occurrence and recurrence. In addition, we cover some culinary controversies that involve certain kinds of fish. We present this information so you can make the choice that's right for you, whether it's obtaining your omegas from wild salmon or relying more on plant sources—flaxseed, canola oil, and walnuts—to get your essential fatty acids.

Bad Fats and Cancer

Structurally, fats are simple molecules built around a series of carbon atoms that are linked together in a chain. Dietary fats are composed of long chains containing twelve to twenty-two carbons. A small change in the structure of a dietary fat can make a big impact on your overall health. Let's first take a look at the fat villains and their role in the cancer process.

Villain: Saturated Fat

Saturated fats are mainly animal fats. They are found in meat, whole-milk dairy products (cheese, milk, and ice cream), and poultry skin. Some plant-based foods, including coconuts and coconut oil, palm oil, and palm kernel oil, are also high in saturated fats. With saturated fatty acids, each of the interior carbon atoms is bonded to two hydrogen atoms as well as two other carbons. All of the bonds available for hydrogen are filled, or "saturated," with hydrogen.

Saturated Fat and Breast Cancer. Data linking saturated fats and cancer are conflicting. Given that saturated fat is a known contributor to heart disease, it is prudent to reduce saturated fat in the diet. Grilled red meat is a source of carcinogens such as heterocyclic amines, *N*-nitroso compounds, and polycyclic aromatic hydrocarbons, which have been found to encourage mammary tumors in animals.

Saturated Fat and Colon Cancer. Similarly, dietary fats have been implicated in the development of colon cancer. Strong evidence exists that red meat—either through its saturated fat content or the cancer-causing compounds produced by cooking meat at high temperatures—promotes colon cancer. Scientists believe that dietary fat increases the excretion of bile acids, which can be converted to carcinogens or promoters. In the 1999 Nurses' Health Study, the risk of colon cancer doubled among women with the highest animal fat intake compared to those with the lowest.

Saturated Fat and Prostate Cancer. The association between fat and prostate cancer has been observed in many studies, although findings have only been consistent for saturated fat. In the Health Professionals Follow-Up Study of 51,000 men, a positive association was seen between intake of red meat, total fat, and animal fat and the risk of prostate cancer. Fats from vegetable sources were unrelated to risk. In some studies, animal fat intake has been most strongly associated with aggressive prostate cancer, suggesting its influence on the transition from a slow-spreading condition to the more lethal form of this cancer.

Healing Tip

By limiting or avoiding red meat and full-fat dairy products, you can minimize your exposure to saturated fat and the cancer-causing agents created when grilling meats. Opt instead for fish, low-fat dairy, and lean poultry—preferably organic or free range.

Villain: Trans Fat

Trans fatty acids are fats produced through a process called *hydrogenation*, which adds a hydrogen to the fat molecule. Hydrogenation became popular because this type of oil doesn't spoil or become rancid as easily as regular oil and therefore has a longer shelf life. The more hydrogenated an oil is, the harder it will be at room temperature. For example, a spreadable tub of margarine is less hydrogenated and so has fewer trans fats than a stick of margarine. Trans fat–free margarine is the best choice. Most of the trans fats in the American diet are found in commercially prepared baked goods, margarines, snack foods, and processed foods, as well as in commercially prepared fried foods, such as french fries and onion rings. A report from the Institute of Medicine concluded that there is no safe level of trans fats in the diet, which prompted the Food and Drug Administration (FDA) to require that all Nutrition Facts food labels list trans fats by January 1, 2006. Check food labels for hydrogenated oils; the higher on the list they appear, the more trans fats there are in the product.

Trans Fats and Cancer. Irrefutably, eating foods containing trans fats increases the risk for heart disease because of the action of these villainous fats on cholesterol; they have also been fingered for their negative impact on blood sugar and insulin—making them evil instigators in the development of diabetes. Similarly, trans fats have an effect on cancer. A recent study conducted at the Health Research Center at the University of Utah showed that postmenopausal women who did not undergo hormone replacement therapy had a twofold increase in risk of colon cancer from high levels of trans fats in their diet. Another timely study conducted by researchers at Harvard found that eating trans fat–containing foods increases *C-reactive protein*, an inflammatory factor most often associated with heart disease and diabetes. However, C-reactive protein, along with other inflammatory factors (called cytokines), are elevated in many forms of cancer.

 Healing Tip

To reduce the inflammatory factors associated with chronic diseases (including cancer), root out trans fat by looking for the terms *partially hydrogenated oils* and *vegetable shortening* on food labels. Choose trans fat–free shortenings and baked goods.

Villain: Fake Fats

The food industry has developed a number of fat substitutes to help consumers reduce their fat consumption. Olestra, also marketed under the misleading name Olean, has been approved by the FDA for use in snacks and fried chips. This fake fat dramatically reduces the absorption of a number of cancer-fighting fat-soluble vitamins and nutrients, which include the carotenoids (beta-carotene, lycopene, and lutein); phytosterols; and vitamins A, E, K, and D.

 Healing Tip

Avoid nutrient-robbing olestra so the precious phytonutrients in your healing whole foods aid in protecting you against cancer occurrence and recurrence.

Good Fats and Cancer

Although it's true that countries with lower average fat intakes tend to have lower rates of breast, colon, and prostate cancers than countries with higher average intakes, closer examination indicates that lifestyle differences—including physical activity, smoking, age at first menstruation, and consumption of fruits and vegetables—are the factors that influence the cancer process. Excess calories and specific *types* of fat rather than the *amount* of fat consumed in the diet also appear to play a role. Let's take a look at the health-promoting fats that benefit insulin function and help to reduce inflammatory processes involved with cancer.

Victor: Monounsaturated Fats

Monounsaturated fats (MUFAs) can be found in vegetable sources, including olives, nuts, and avocados. The double bond allows the monounsaturated fatty acid chain to be a bit more fluid, making them liquid at room temperature.

Like their cousins, the polyunsaturated fats (PUFAs), monounsaturated fats are best known for their ability to decrease blood cholesterol levels as part of a healthful diet. They have also been found to contribute to glycemic control, helping to keep blood sugar stable, and decrease the risk of heart disease, diabetes, and possibly cancer. We will discuss in Chapter 5 how compounds in foods team up to protect our health, a phenomenon called *synergy*.

Monounsaturated Fat and Breast Cancer. Studies conducted in Spain and Greece have shown the protective effect of monounsaturated fats, particularly olive oil, against breast cancer. Researchers believe the antioxidants, specifically phenolic compounds, and relatively high content of monounsaturated fat are responsible for these effects.

Monounsaturated Fat and Prostate Cancer. A recent UCLA study found similar results for prostate cancer. Researchers looked at the cancer-preventive effects of California Haas avocados on prostate cells. In test-tube studies they found that compounds in avocados—including MUFAs, carotenoids such as lutein, and tocopherols—inhibited the growth of prostate cancer cells. However, when lutein alone was tested, no such effect was seen, suggesting again that these fat-soluble nutrients buddy up with MUFAs to decrease cancer risk.

Monounsaturated Fat and Colon Cancer. A recent Swiss study found an inverse association between colon cancer risk and the consumption of monounsaturated fat.

Although less research exists for the role of MUFAs and colon cancer, we know choosing this good fat over the villainous ones described previously can do a lot to protect the health of your heart and to balance your blood sugar.

 Kitchen Prescription

Stock your kitchen with nuts, nonhydrogenated nut butters, olive oil, and avocados to get the benefits of health-promoting MUFAs. Trade in your chips and pretzels for a MUFA-rich snack mix that includes popcorn popped in canola oil and raw almonds

Victor: Polyunsaturated Fats

The human body needs fatty acids and can make all but two of them: linolenic and linoleic acid. These fats must be supplied by the diet; hence the term *essential fatty acids* (*EFA*s). Used by the body to maintain cell membranes and make hormonelike substances that regulate blood pressure, clotting, immune response, insulin function, and blood lipids, the PUFA side of the fat family gets special treatment for its good behavior and positive impact on health.

Omega-3 fatty acids, also known as *linolenic acid*, are essential fatty acids that come from both plant and animal sources. When given linolenic acid, the body can make *eicosapentaenoic acid* (*EPA*) and *docosahexaenoic acid* (*DHA*), the two major fatty acids in fish. The greatest amounts of EPA and DHA are found in oily, dark-fleshed fish that live in deep, cold waters such as tuna, bluefish, and salmon. *Alpha-linolenic acid* is the other essential fatty acid and is found most abundantly in canola oil (11 percent), as well as in flaxseed and walnuts. Soybeans also contain a balance of omega-3 fats.

Omega-6 fatty acids also known as *linoleic acid*, are much more common in the American diet and are found in soybean oil, safflower oil, sunflower oil, corn oil, wheat germ, and sesame.

Let's take a look at each of the essentials and their role in cancer prevention and treatment.

Omega-3 Fats and Cancer. Long known to protect the heart, omega-3s also positively influence inflammatory processes, cell communication, and how genes make proteins. Because of this, they have been the target of much attention for their role in preventing and treating cancer.

Studies have shown that the omega-3 fatty acids are involved in cell signaling and help cause cancer cells to self-destruct, a process called *apoptosis*. A 2004 study published in the *International Journal of Cancer* showed that omega-3s stopped the growth of cancer in test-tube and animal studies and improve the function of the liver and pancreas in postoperative cancer patients.

Omega-3s are also useful in cancer therapy. A recent study conducted at Louisiana State University found that the effects of cancer drugs—including doxorubicin, 5-fluorouracil, epirubicin, CPT-11, and tamoxifen—and radiation therapy have been improved when patients' diets included omega-3 fatty acids. The consumption of omega-3s was also found to produce more positive treatment outcomes and the potential to slow or prevent the recurrence of cancer.

Omega-6 Fats and Cancer. While omega-6 fatty acids are "good" fats, there is a dark side to these acids that has been created by modern technology. Snacks and most foods we consume tend to be high in omega-6s, which when left unbalanced by their anti-inflammatory counterpart omega-3, can lead to health problems, including cardiovascular disease, cancer, and inflammatory and autoimmune diseases.

A recent study conducted at The Center for Genetics Nutrition and Health found that a 2:1 ratio of omega-3 to omega-6 reduced cancer cell proliferation in patients with colorectal cancer, and a lower omega-6 to omega-3 ratio in women with breast cancer decreased risk.

The important thing to remember is to strive for a good balance of omega-3 to omega-6, which can be achieved by consuming more whole foods and following some of our practical tips.

Kitchen Prescription

To improve your omega-3 to omega-6 ratio, try the following:

+ Choose canola oil when cooking.
+ Select walnuts as a snack.
+ Look for new food products, including eggs, breads, and cereals, with enhanced omega-3s.
+ Try flaxseed meal or hempseed meal as an addition to smoothies, cereals, and baked goods.
+ Include cold-water fish such as salmon and tuna in your diet. Learn more about choosing fish in the following section.

The Dish on Fish. As we've already discussed, there are numerous benefits to the omega-3 fatty acids in fish. Although there is no doubt that including fish in your diet will deliver cancer-protective essential fatty acids and B vitamins, recent studies show that there are different schools of thought when it comes to what fish you choose.

Although farm-raising salmon allows more fish to get to market at an affordable price and ultimately end up on our tables, recent controversy has made some people concerned as to whether farm-raised salmon is contaminated by cancer-causing industrial chemicals. If you choose to consume farmed salmon score the flesh, grill or broil salmon to 175°F, allow the juices to run off, and remove the skin. This could reduce harmful contaminants by half.

Research also shows that certain types of fish may contain dangerous levels of mercury. Nearly all fish and shellfish contain traces of *methylmercury*, a type of mercury found in water that can be harmful, especially to unborn babies and young children whose nervous systems are still developing. The risk for mercury lies in both the type of seafood consumed and the amount. In a joint consumer advisory, the Food and Drug Administration and the Environmental Protection Agency warn that women who are trying to become pregnant, pregnant women, nursing mothers, and young children should avoid the types of fish and shellfish with higher levels of mercury and eat only those with lower levels. If you regularly eat fish high in methylmercury, the substance can accumulate in your blood over time. Although it is removed from the body naturally, it may take more than a year for the levels to drop significantly, which is why women who are trying to become pregnant should avoid eating certain types of fish.

In addition to the known negative health consequences of mercury, its role in cancer has also been explored. In animal studies, mercury has been found to cause tumors and promote cancer. A recent study published in *Environmental Toxicology* (2005) found that methylmercury stimulates the growth of breast cancer cells, although much more research in this area is needed to understand the mechanisms.

While almost all fish and shellfish contain traces of methylmercury, larger fish that have lived longer contain the highest levels because the element accumulates over time. Avoid eating shark, swordfish, king mackerel, or tilefish because they contain high levels of mercury and pose the greatest risk. You should be eating up to twelve ounces (two average meals) a week of a variety of fish and shellfish that are lower in mercury. We offer several recipes that include fish in Chapter 9. Five of the most commonly eaten fish that are low in mercury are shrimp, canned light tuna, salmon, pollack, and catfish. Albacore (white) tuna has more mercury than canned light tuna. When choosing your two meals of fish and shellfish, you may eat up to six ounces, one average meal, of albacore tuna per week. In addition, you should check to see whether advisories exist concerning the safety of fish caught in local lakes, rivers, and coastal areas. If no advice is available, eat up to six ounces per week of fish you catch from local waters.

What Are Carbohydrates?

Carbohydrates are produced by photosynthesis in plants and are the primary source of energy found in plants, including fruits, vegetables, grains, legumes, and tubers. Carbohydrates have an important role in the function of our internal organs, nervous system, and muscles, and they are the best source of energy for endurance athletics because they provide both immediate and time-released energy. These compounds are needed to regulate protein and fat metabolism, as well as to help fight infections, promote growth, and lubricate the joints.

Traditionally, carbs have been grouped into two main categories: simple carbs, which include sugars such as fruit sugar (fructose), corn or grape sugar (dextrose or glucose), and table sugar (sucrose); and complex carbs, which include everything made of three or more linked sugars. In the digestive system, carbohydrates are broken down into single sugar molecules, which are then absorbed into the bloodstream and used as energy.

Not All Carbs Are Created Equal

It's a shame that the entire carbohydrate family gets a bad rap for their delinquent stripped cousins. The naked truth of the matter is that when the integrity of whole grains is preserved, the effects on health are nothing short of wholesome.

Traditionally, it has been assumed that complex carbohydrates cause smaller rises in blood sugar than do simple carbohydrates. A growing body of evidence, however, contradicts this notion. In fact, white bread and potatoes are digested almost immediately to glucose, causing blood sugar to spike rapidly—refuting the theory that complex carbohydrates are different from simple sugars in terms of their effects on blood sugar levels. A new system that has been embraced by some in the scientific community, called the *glycemic index (GI)*, rates foods according to how fast and how far they push blood sugar, giving us a better indication of how carb-rich foods affect health.

It has been shown that the GI of a food depends on the speed of digestion and absorption into the body, which is largely determined by both its physical and chemical properties. Typically, foods with less starch to gelatinize (such as pasta) and those containing a high level of soluble fiber (such as whole-grain barley, oats, and rye) have slower rates of digestion and lower GI values. Another important influence on GI values is the ratio of a compound called *amylose* to a fiber called *amylopectin*. Foods with a higher amylose-amylopectin ratio, such as legumes and parboiled rice, tend to have lower GI values due to the compact structure of amylose, which blunts the effects of enzymatic reactions. Conversely, amylopectin is a branched compound, making it more available to enzymatic attack in the body and promoting digestion. Use of the glycemic index has shown that many complex carbohydrates (like the white bread and potatoes already noted) cause endocrine responses that rival pure glucose, further casting doubt on the usefulness of the simple versus complex classification system.

The principal argument against the GI concept is that it cannot tell the entire story, because blood sugar levels are influenced by both the quantity and the quality (GI rating) of the carbohydrate. In response to this concern, the concept of glycemic load (GL) was introduced. Defined as the product of the GI value of a food and its carbohydrate content, GL incorporates both the quality and quantity of carbohydrate consumed.

In quantifying the glucose-raising potential of dietary carbohydrates, each unit of glycemic load is equivalent to 1 gram of carbohydrate from white bread. In general, carbohydrate-dense foods with low fiber content, including potatoes, refined cereal products, and many sugar-sweetened beverages, have high GI and GL values, whereas whole grains, fruits, and vegetables with high fiber content provide low to very low GLs per serving. It should be noted, however, that many low-GI foods are not necessarily high in fiber (for example, pasta, basmati rice, and dairy products), whereas some high-fiber, whole-meal bread and cereal products are high in GI.

Valuable research in recent years has offered additional insight into how carbohydrates affect our endocrine system, including insulin and sex hormones and their influence on cancer processes, as well as hunger, overeating, and weight gain.

Refined Versus Whole Carbohydrates: Messing with Mother Nature. When it became a common practice to refine the wheat flour for bread by milling it and discarding the bran and germ, consumers lost a myriad of health-protective nutrients. In the 1940s, Congress passed legislation requiring that all grain products crossing state lines be enriched with iron, thiamin, riboflavin, and niacin. In 1996, this legislation was amended to include folate, because of its important role in preventing birth defects. Although enrichment—the process of adding nutrients to a food to meet a specific standard—restores and raises many of the nutrients lost during refining, recent research shows that the health consequences cannot be compensated for by adding individual nutrients back to a refined grain product for several reasons.

First, by removing the germ and bran layers of a grain, a naturally low-GI food is turned into one with a high GI. The fibrous coating serves to slow digestion, keeping blood sugar on an even keel. Also, the surface area is increased with refined grain products, enhancing digestive enzyme processes. As we discussed previously, this is an important element in keeping insulin and insulin-like growth factor (IGF) levels low and in maintaining a healthy weight.

Second, many nutrients in the germ and bran layers are not added back to the refined grain product, or the body can't absorb them well. This is especially true of minerals, which are not as well absorbed from enriched foods as from natural sources. Magnesium, which has an important role in insulin function, and zinc, a mineral important for a healthy immune system, are two to note.

Third, the "new nutritional frontier" is still in its infancy, and we have yet to identify all of the health-protective compounds in every food. When we alter a food from its natural state—by refining, for example—we may be removing a cocktail of phytonutrients and other compounds that protect us from disease.

Numerous studies have shown that consuming whole grains reduces the risk of cancers, including those of the gastrointestinal tract (mouth, stomach, and colon) and hormonally dependent cancers (including breast and prostate).

Carbohydrate Choices and Cancer Risk

Research shows that choosing high-GI carbohydrates elevates insulin and stimulates cancer-promoting IGFs. Although research is ongoing, numerous studies postulate an association between IGFs and several forms of cancer. In the Women's Health Study of 39,876 women followed for eight years, positive associations were found between dietary glycemic load, overall glycemic index, and the risk of colorectal cancer in women, although other studies have found no association or have been inconclusive.

Insulin-like growth factors are also being examined for their role in prostate cancer. Investigators from the Harvard School of Public Health, the Karolinska Institute of Stockholm, and the University of Athens studied 150 Greek men to evaluate the role of hormones in prostate disease. The study found that men with higher levels of IGF-1 had a higher risk of developing prostate cancer but not benign prostatic hyperplasia (BPH). A more recent study involving more than 2,500 Italian men bolstered this evidence, showing a direct relation between dietary GI and GL and prostate cancer risk.

The Nurses' Health Study II examined carbohydrates in the diet, glycemic load, and fiber in relation to the risk of breast cancer among 90,655 women. Although carbohydrate in the diet, glycemic load, and glycemic index were not related to breast cancer in the overall study, an association and an increased risk were found for women with a body mass index (BMI) of 25 or higher. This study also investigated the effects of diet during high school on the risk of breast cancer as an adult. Using a retrospective food frequency questionnaire, researchers interviewed 47,355 women and found that a higher dietary glycemic index during adolescence was associated with an increased risk of breast cancer.

Carbohydrate Choices and Cancer Treatment

Because of their high fiber and water content, whole-grain foods contain fewer calories per gram than the same amount of corresponding refined-grain food. The Nurses' Health Study showed that women with the greatest increased intake of whole grains gained an average of 1.52 kilograms less than did those with the smallest increase in intake. In addition, women with the highest consumption of whole grains had a 49 percent lower risk of major weight gain than did women with the highest consumption of refined grains. Researchers believe that the insulin-elevating effects of high-GI foods promotes weight gain by directing nutrients away from use by muscles and toward storage in fat cells.

Because foods high on the glycemic index elevate insulin and promote development of IGFs and inflammation, there is good reason to avoid refined carbohydrates if you have cancer. Although additional research is needed to clarify the role of the glycemic index in these diseases, almost every study conducted on the effects of carbohydrates on appetite has shown that low-GI foods produce a feeling of satiety, or satisfaction, for a longer period of time than do their high-GI counterparts. One study found both lower levels of blood sugar and a slower return of hunger after meals with a bean-based dish (low GI) versus a potato dish (high GI). Because evidence supports the theory that low-GI carbohydrates promote satiety and reduce overeating—both of which contribute to achieving or maintaining a healthy weight—limiting these foods could be a key factor for cancer prevention and recurrence.

Carbs in the Kitchen

Now that we've set the stage for understanding how carbohydrates affect the cancer process, let's put it into practice. Here we offer information on classifying carbs, show you how easy it is to clean up your carb act, and give you practical pairings to get your good carbs and good fats deliciously.

Classifying Carbs

While certain fruits and vegetables, like watermelon and carrots, are high on the GI scale, they should not be avoided because they have an abundance of phytonutrients, fiber, and other nutrients and carrots have a low GL. Aim to stock your pantry with low-GI foods, and enjoy them often. Look at Tables 3.1 through 3.3 to start stocking up on an appropriate balance of high-, moderate-, and low-GI foods.

Clean Up Your Carb Act

Small changes can make a big impact on your health. The list that follows Table 3.2 offers some helpful suggestions for replacing the carbs higher on the glycemic index with some healthier alternatives.

TABLE 3.1 **Foods with a High Glycemic Index (Greater than 69)**	
Product	**Food**
Breads and bakery	White bread
	Whole-meal bread
	Pretzels
	French bread
Breakfast cereals	Corn Flakes
	Rice Krispies
	Cheerios
Confectionery	Jelly beans
	LifeSavers
	Skittles
Fruits and vegetables	Carrots
	Watermelon
	Potatoes
	Parsnips
Rice, grains, and pastas	Low-amylase rice

TABLE 3.2 **Foods with a Moderate Glycemic Index (55–69)**	
Product	**Food**
Breads and bakery	Sourdough
	Pita bread
	Barley bread
	Rye bread
	Whole-wheat bread
Breakfast cereals	Quick-cooking oatmeal
	Cream of Wheat
	Muesli
Dairy foods	Ice cream, full fat
Fruits and vegetables	Pineapple
	Popcorn
	Pawpaw
Rice, grains, and pastas	Brown rice
	Linguine
	White rice

❖ Instead of white bread, try pumpernickel or whole-grain breads.
❖ Instead of white rice, try basmati rice or Lundberg rice.
❖ Instead of sugary breakfast cereal, try muesli, steel-cut oats, or All Bran.
❖ Instead of pretzels, try popcorn.
❖ Instead of potatoes, try beans or whole-wheat pasta.
❖ Instead of white crackers, try rye crisps.
❖ Instead of cakes, light muffins, or pastries, try bran muffins or whole-grain mixes.

TABLE 3.3 Foods with a Low Glycemic Index (Less than 55)

Product	Food
Breads and bakery	Pumpernickel
	Heavy mixed grain
Breakfast cereals	All Bran
	Toasted muesli
	Psyllium-based cereal
	Oatmeal (old-fashioned)
Dairy foods	Milk, full fat
	Soy milk
	Milk, skim
	Yogurt, low fat, fruit
Fruits and vegetables	Grapefruit
	Peach
	Apple
	Pear
	Orange
	Grapes
	Kiwi
	Banana
	Sweet potato
Rice, grains, and pastas	Fettuccini
	Whole-wheat spaghetti
	Spaghetti
	Long-grain rice
	Bulgur
Legumes	Peanuts
	Soybeans
	Lentils
	Chickpeas
	Baked beans (canned)

Perfect Pairings

Here are some ideas from Healing Gourmet on getting a daily dose of those good fats and good carbs with no sacrifice in taste. For more ideas on perfect pairings for balanced health, see the recipe and meal planning sections, and visit our website at healing gourmet.com.

- ❖ Pepperidge Farm German Dark Wheat Toast with all-natural peanut butter for whole grains, PUFAs, and low-GI legumes
- ❖ Ryvita Dark Rye crackers and hummus for whole grains, low-GI legumes, and MUFAs
- ❖ Grilled wild salmon and Lundberg Wehani Rice for whole grains and omega-3s
- ❖ Stonyfield Farms black cherry yogurt and ground flax for low-GI carbs and omega-3s

Now that you have some ideas for balancing the good and bad fats and carbohydrates, it's time to look at the benefits of increasing your intake of antioxidants and phytonutrients, as well as ways to incorporate these important foods into your diet.

Antioxidants, Phytonutrients, and Other Cancer- Fighting Nutrients

INDIVIDUAL COMPOUNDS in foods get special attention for their honorable actions as defenders of our health. These antioxidant nutrients and phytonutrients join forces to keep our cells healthy and prevent the DNA damage that can lead to cancer. As these nutrients work in a team, no single nutrient has the ability to conquer disease. In this chapter we'll discuss the lineup of nutrients and phytonutrients that play a role in a cancer-fighting nutritional strategy.

Free Radical Defense

In the fight against cancer, the free radical opposition makes about ten thousand attacks every day. These unstable oxygen molecules have lost an electron and, like a sneaky opponent, move swiftly through the playing field of your body, trying to steal electrons from other molecules. This in turn creates more free radicals and leaves damaged cells behind. Some free radicals arise normally during metabolism, but environmental factors such as pollution, poor food choices, radiation, cigarette smoke, and herbicides can also generate them.

Our body's defense, including the immune system and antioxidants produced by the liver (such as glutathione and superoxide dismutase), needs fuel from outside sources to stave off our cancerous adversary. Quite simply, the fuel is food, and good dietary decisions tip the odds in favor of our health.

Phytonutrient Fuel

Inside plants—including the fruits, vegetables, legumes, and grains we eat—there are compounds called *phytonutrients* (*phyto* means "plant") that protect against harsh weather conditions and hungry insects. These compounds even heal the wounds made by nibbling moths. With their own defensive lineup, plants stand ready to guard against hungry predators that try to take a bite or fungi that hang around and drain their resources.

This plant protection system—essentially antioxidants and phytonutrients—not only serve as a defense but are also responsible for the vibrant colors and delicious flavors of our food. Interestingly, the ability to distinguish color is a trait common only to humans and a few species of primates. So the foods that are most appealing to our eye are also most appealing to our body to prevent and treat diseases, including cancer.

It should come as no surprise that fruits and vegetables with higher levels of antioxidants remain fresh for longer periods of time (shelf life) with less risk of mold. These foods are better equipped to preserve and protect themselves; and when we take a bite, we become the receivers of the powerful antioxidants and phytonutrients—passing on a bevy of cancer-fighting nutrients on to us.

Unfortunately, the development of agriculture some ten thousand years ago caused a shift away from the diverse, plant-based diet that provided a spectrum of essential vitamins and minerals as well as tens of thousands of protective phytonutrients.

Replacing this delicious and defensive diet with processed foods, refined grains, added oils, sugar, and salt has led to the rise of chronic diseases, including cancer. In fact, today most Americans eat between two and three servings of fruits and vegetables per day (when the optimum is seven to nine servings), and some people eat none at all.

Advances in technology have allowed us to further explore compounds in foods on a molecular level, distinguishing between the thousands of plant nutrients in individual foods and food families. This "new nutritional frontier" provides us with critical information on how we can best use foods to protect us from cancer and even regain our health.

It is estimated that twenty-five thousand individual phytonutrients have been identified in fruits, vegetables, and grains; but a large percentage still remain unknown and need to be identified before we can fully understand their health benefits.

Your body's defense system is assisted by the phytonutrient fuel you feed it. Each time you eat fruits, vegetables, or other antioxidant-rich foods a flood of anticancer nutrients enters your bloodstream to protect and repair your DNA, starve cancer cells, and promote well-being. Let's take a look at the team of nutrients working together for your health.

Vitamins, Minerals, and Cancer

These old-school standbys have taught us a few new things in recent decades. Although we have known about the actions of vitamins and minerals for some time, it is only recently that we have begun to understand their individual roles in cancer. See Table 4.1 for information on serving sizes.

Folate

Folate gets its name from the Latin word *folium* for "leaf" and is present in large amounts in leafy greens. Folate works in con-

TABLE 4.1 Serving Size Guide

Food Group	Serving Size	Visual Comparison
Grains	1 slice bread; ½ cup cooked cereal, rice, or pasta; 1 cup ready-to-eat cereal	½ cup cooked pasta = a scoop of ice cream; 1 cup dry cereal = a large handful
Vegetables	½ cup chopped raw or cooked veggies; 1 cup leafy raw veggies	1 cup veggies = the size of your fist
Fruits	1 medium apple, orange, or banana; ½ cup juice or canned fruit; ¼ cup dried fruit	1 medium piece of fruit = a baseball
Dairy	1 cup milk or yogurt; 2 ounces cheese	2 ounces cheese = a pair of dominos
Protein foods	3 ounces cooked lean meat, poultry, or fish; ½ cup dried beans, 1 egg counts as 1 ounce of lean meat; 2 tablespoons peanut butter	3 ounces meat or fish = the palm of your hand
Fats	1 teaspoon butter; 1 teaspoon oil	1 teaspoon butter = the tip of your thumb

junction with vitamin B_6 and vitamin B_{12}. Many studies have shown that people who get more folate in their diets have a reduced risk of colon, rectal, and breast cancers.

Folate seems to be of particular importance for people who consume alcohol.

Numerous studies have found that even moderate alcohol intake is associated with an increased risk of breast cancer in women. However, in those women who consume at least one alcoholic drink per day, a folic acid intake of at least 600 micrograms daily resulted in about half the risk of breast cancer compared with women who consumed less than 300 micrograms.

Studies have also found that low folate intake and high alcohol intake are associated with an increased risk of colorectal cancer. In a study of more than forty-five thousand male health professionals, the intake of more than two alcoholic drinks per day doubled the risk of colon cancer. The combination of high alcohol and low folate intake increased the risk of colon cancer further. However, among those in the two-cocktail-a-day group, the men who took 650 micrograms or more of folate per day negated that increased risk.

 Kitchen Prescription

Beans and Greens! If you frequently dine on "beans and greens," you're fine with folate. If you imbibe (which should be done in moderation), pay close attention to this vitamin and dip up a second helping of folate-rich green foods. You can get it in black-eyed peas (105 mcg or 25% DV), cooked spinach (100 mcg or 25% DV), great northern beans (90 mcg or 20% DV), asparagus (85 mcg or 20% DV), wheat germ (40 mcg or 10% DV), orange juice (35 mcg or 10% DV), peas (50 mcg or 15%), cooked broccoli (45 mcg or 15%), avocado (45 mcg or 10% DV), and peanuts (40 mcg or 10% DV).

Vitamin B$_6$

Vitamin B$_6$ is a water-soluble vitamin that performs a wide variety of functions in your body and is essential for good health. It is needed for more than one hundred enzymes involved in protein metabolism and is essential for red blood cell metabolism. The nervous and immune systems require vitamin B$_6$ to function efficiently, and it is also needed for the conversion of tryptophan (an amino acid) to niacin (a vitamin).

In association with the research on folate and cancer, vitamin B$_6$ has been evaluated for its role in reducing cancer risk. A recent study conducted at Harvard's Division of Preventive Medicine found that higher levels of vitamin B$_6$ in the body may reduce the risk of developing breast cancer.

Scientists believe that the combination of folate, vitamin B$_6$, and vitamin B$_{12}$ works to preserve and repair DNA for protection against cancer occurrence and recurrence.

 Kitchen Prescription

Don't Nix the Six! You can find vitamin B$_6$ in potatoes (0.7 mg or 35% DV), garbanzo beans (0.57 mg or 30% DV), chicken breast (0.52 mg or 25% DV), oatmeal (0.42 mg or 20% DV), trout (0.29 mg or 15% DV), sunflower seeds (0.23 mg or 10% DV), avocado (0.20 mg or 10% DV), tuna (0.18 mg or 10% DV), and cooked spinach (0.14 mg or 8% DV).

Vitamin B$_{12}$

Vitamin B$_{12}$ is also called cobalamin. It is bound to the protein in food and is released by hydrochloric acid (HCl) in the stomach during digestion. Vitamin B$_{12}$ is needed for normal nerve activity, is necessary for DNA replication, and is important for the formation of red blood cells. Two prospective studies—the Nurses' Health Study and one in Washington County, Maryland—found a relationship between low vitamin B_{12} and an increased risk of breast cancer.

 Kitchen Prescription

Go Fish! Vitamin B_{12} is found in clams (84.1 mcg or 1,400% DV), trout (5.4 mcg or 90% DV), salmon (4.9 mcg or 80% DV), yogurt (1.4 mcg or 25% DV), tuna (1 mcg or 15% DV), and milk (0.9 mcg or 15% DV).

Vitamin C

Vitamin C is a water-soluble vitamin that's also known as ascorbic acid. This vitamin is involved in collagen synthesis, wound healing, infection resistance, and iron absorption; it's also an antioxidant. The recommended daily allowance (RDA) for smokers is higher than that for nonsmokers, because smokers are under increased oxidative stress from the toxins in cigarette smoke and generally have lower blood levels of vitamin C. Dr. Linus Pauling made the use of vitamin C for cancer therapy popular. In addition, researchers now know that vitamin C, like every other team player, works in synergy with other nutrient teammates to protect against cancer.

 Kitchen Prescription

Orange You Healthy? Get your daily dose of vitamin C in citrus fruits, berries, mangoes, papaya, melons, tomatoes, sweet potatoes, peppers, and green leafy vegetables.

Vitamin D

This fat-soluble vitamin helps to maintain normal blood levels of calcium and phosphorus, aids in the absorption of calcium from food, promotes bone mineralization, and reduces the loss of calcium from the body. In addition, it is necessary for healthy bones and teeth and may help reduce the risk of cancer. The body converts vitamin D from foods or sunlight into a hormonal form that has cancer-fighting activity. This form—25-hydroxyvitamin D, or 25(OH)D—has been shown to halt the growth of colon, prostate, and pancreatic cancer cells in the lab. A recent Harvard review of the current evidence on the role of vitamins in the risk, prevention, and treatment of breast cancer found an inverse association between vitamin D and breast cancer risk, although more studies are needed.

 Kitchen Prescription

"D-lightful" Foods! Get a dose of D with salmon (360 IU or 90% DV), mackerel (345 IU or 90% DV), sardines (250 IU or 70% DV), tuna (200 IU or 50% DV), and milk (98 IU or 25% DV).

Vitamin E

This fat-soluble vitamin exists in eight different forms, each having its own biological activity. *Alpha-tocopherol* is the most active form in humans and is a strong antioxidant. Not only does it protect cells from the effects of free radicals, but it also enhances immune function and blocks the formation of nitrosamines, which are carcinogens formed in the stomach from nitrites consumed in the diet.

Kitchen Prescription

Es to Please! Vitamin E is found in wheat germ oil (20.3 mg or 100% DV), almonds (7.4 mg or 40% DV), sunflower seeds (6 mg or 40% DV), hazelnuts (4.3 mg or 20% DV), peanuts (2.2 mg or 10% DV), mango (0.9 mg or 6% DV), broccoli (1.2 mg or 6% DV), spinach (1.6 mg or 6% DV), and kiwi (1.1 mg or 6% DV).

Selenium

Although selenium is a mineral rather than a nutrient, it is a component of antioxidant enzymes. The amount of selenium in soil, which varies by region, determines the amount of selenium in the foods grown in that soil. Scientists have explored selenium's role in cancer as an important part of antioxidant enzymes that protect cells against the effects of free radicals produced during normal metabolism.

Studies show that selenium may help cancer cells self-destruct (a process called apoptosis), improve the function of the immune system (specifically natural killer cells), and reduce the rate of tumor growth. Selenium appears to have a special role in protecting men from prostate cancer.

Kitchen Prescription

Go Nuts! Brazil nuts contain large quantities of selenium (540 mg or 780% DV). You can also find it in tuna (63 mg or 95% DV), cod (32 mg or 45% DV), turkey (32 mg or 45% DV), chicken (20 mg or 30% DV), noodles (17 mg or 25% DV), and oatmeal (12 mg or 15% DV).

The Phytonutrient Team of Players

Don't let the big names of these tiny compounds scare you. They deliver a powerful punch, even when you don't call them by name. The important thing is to remember to include the full spectrum of cancer-fighting phytonutrients in your diet every day!

Phenolic Phytonutrients and Flavonoids

Phenolics represent a very large category of more than two thousand phytonutrients. The term *phenol* comes from the chemical structure of these phytonutrients, which varies from one to several phenol groups. These powerful groups have the ability to sweep up many free radicals as they circulate through the bloodstream, rendering those cancer-causing scoundrels harmless. Considered to be some of the most powerful antioxidants, phenolics are being studied for their ability to slow the aging process and also have anti-inflammatory, clot-busting, tumor-fighting, and heart-protective effects. Let's take a look at the phenolic family and how each member allies forces for your health.

Flavonoids. These are molecular compounds found only in plants, which serve as a defense mechanism. Because plants don't have the fight-or-flight option of animals, they must protect themselves chemically; flavonoids make the plant tissue unappetizing to fungi, insects, and other harmful organisms. Every plant makes flavonoids, but they tend to be concentrated in leaves and fruit. For that reason, fruits tend to be a richer source of flavonoids than many vegetables. Dietary flavonoids have been found to repair a range of oxidative radical damage to DNA, which can contribute to disease and the ravages of aging.

Kitchen Prescription

Fabulous flavonoids can be found in apples, broccoli, celery, citrus fruits, cocoa, eggplant, endive, grapes, grapefruit, leeks, onion, parsley, raspberries, red wine, strawberries, and tea.

Tannins. These substances, primarily found in tea, have been studied for their action on inflammation and their ability to kill viruses and bacteria. Lab studies also show that tannins halt the formation of skin cancer in animal studies and help colon cancer cells to self-destruct.

 Kitchen Prescription

Drink to Your Health! Get tannins in oolong tea, black tea, sorghum, red wine, and coffee.

Epigallocatechin gallate (EGCG). This polyphenol comes primarily from green tea. It has antioxidant activity and has been found to have a wide range of health-promoting benefits, from reducing allergies to helping prevent and reverse the cancer process. Researchers at the University of Alabama's Clinical Nutrition Research Center found that EGCG has the ability to prevent breast cancer as well as its spread (metastasis) by helping cancer cells self-destruct.

 Kitchen Prescription

Make a Cancer-Fighting Cocktail! Steep 4 green tea bags, preferably organic, in 4 cups of hot spring water for 3 minutes. Add fresh mint leaves, and allow to cool. Pour into a pitcher and refrigerate for a delicious drink—with EGCG benefits.

Anthocyanins. These brightly colored compounds have recently been found to protect against cancer through multiple actions. In the lab, they halt the mutations that change normal cells into cancerous ones, cause apoptosis, and reduce inflammatory processes related to cancer.

Research also shows that anthocyanins may inhibit the growth of cancer. Cancer forms new blood vessels that act as nutrient superhighways to feed it. This process, called *angiogenesis* (*angio* meaning "blood vessel," and *genesis* meaning "new"), may be decreased by these amazing berry phytonutrients. A recent study conducted at the Bioactive Natural Products and Phytoceuticals Department of Michigan State reports that anthocyanins also stop the growth of existing cancer.

 Kitchen Prescription

Berry Delicious Medicine! You can find these compounds most readily in red-blue fruits and vegetables, including blueberries, raspberries, lingonberries, cherries, currants, pomegranate, strawberries, Concord grapes, cranberries, and elderberries. Buy them frozen and add them to smoothies or thaw for a quick addition to cereal.

Quercetin. This naturally occurring antioxidant helps fight cancer, protects the heart, and slows the effects of aging. Studies have shown that quercetin may halt the growth of skin and colon cancer and (like anthocyanins) induce apoptosis—or cell suicide—in breast and prostate cancer cells. It may also reduce the risk of lung cancer, especially in men.

 Kitchen Prescription

Don't Quit the Quercetin! You can get quercetin in red grapes, red and yellow onions, broccoli, and apples.

Kaempferol. This nutrient has been found to cause apoptosis in prostate and breast cancer cell cultures in the laboratory.

 Kitchen Prescription

Cancer-Killing Kaempferol! You will find this antioxidant in broccoli as well as grapefruit, leeks, and strawberries.

Isoflavones. Isoflavones are *phytoestrogens* (plant estrogens) that interfere with estrogen's ability to interact with and encourage the growth of certain tumor cells. Certain types of tumors need estrogen in order to grow. But the estrogen can't promote tumor growth unless it can "park" in specific estrogen receptors on tumor cells. Isoflavones can prevent the tumors from growing by inserting themselves into the receptor "parking spaces," leaving no place for the estrogen. There are numerous isoflavones, including diadzein, genistein, and glycitein.

 Kitchen Prescription

Phyte Cancer! You can find these phytoestrogens in soy, beans, peas, lentils, and mushrooms.

Ellagic Acid. Ellagic acid has been found to inhibit mutations and exhibits anticarcinogenic activity by disarming carcinogens before they can make healthy cells cancerous.

 Kitchen Prescription

Strategic Ellagic! Get this phenolic compound in strawberries, grapes, and cherries.

Curcumin. Credited for the unique flavors and golden color of curries, curcumin has potent antioxidant activity and has been found to help prevent and halt cancer. Research shows that this spicy phytonutrient helps to prevent the cell mutations that lead to cancer, causes cancer cells to self-destruct, and prevents the formation of new blood vessels to the tumor.

Studies have also shown that, because of these actions, curcumin has therapeutic potential in assisting in the recovery from breast, colon, and prostate cancers.

 Kitchen Prescription

Spicy Protection! Curcumin is found in turmeric, and you can get the benefits of this amazing phytonutrient with our recipe for Indian Spice Mix.

Indian Spice Mix

2 teaspoons ground turmeric	8 teaspoons dry mustard
4 teaspoons ground fenugreek	4 teaspoons ground cumin
2 teaspoons ground ginger	2 teaspoons ground coriander
2 teaspoons ground cloves	½ teaspoon ground cinnamon

Combine all ingredients in a small bowl with an airtight lid. Shake well to blend. Store in a cool dry place, sealed. Add the mixture to chicken, fish, and bean dishes.

Makes about 24½ teaspoons

Gingerols. These aromatic phytonutrients are found in—what else?—ginger! This compound and others in the ginger family have been found to stop the growth and division of cancer cells by causing apoptosis, or cell suicide.

Kitchen Prescription

Add Some Zing! Ginger is a member of the Zingiberaceae family, which also includes turmeric. Get it in our Tummy-Soothing Smoothie.

Ferulic Acid. This antioxidant phytonutrient is present mainly in grains. It was found to halt the formation of colon cancer in studies conducted at the Department of Pathology, Gifu University School of Medicine, Japan.

Kitchen Prescription

Great Grains! Get ferulic acid in whole-grain foods, which also stabilize blood sugar and give you a healthy dose of fiber.

Lentinan. A compound found mainly in shiitake mushrooms, this phytonutrient stimulates the production and action of immune cells, including natural killer cells and macrophages, which destroy tumor cells.

Kitchen Prescription

Fabulous Fungus! Try our Shiitake-and-Rappini-Stuffed Chicken Breasts for a healthy dose of this cancer fighter.

Resveratrol. This substance, found in the skins of red and white grapes, grape juice, and red wine, exhibits anticancer activity in the laboratory. It is not found in white wine because the grape skin—which contains the resveratrol—is discarded early in the manufacturing process.

Kitchen Prescription

Grape Protection! Try different varieties of grapes and always wash well. Better yet, try organic varieties that have been grown without the use of pesticides.

Hesperetin. In combination with other citrus compounds, hesperetin has been found to protect against cancers of the colon and breast. As part of a "flavonoid cocktail" tested at the University of Buffalo, in test tubes, hesperetin helped to kill breast cancer cells that had become resistant to drug treatment.

Similarly, a study conducted at the University of Western Ontario showed that hesperetin-rich orange juice given to breast cancer patients enhanced the cancer-crushing effects of tamoxifen, showing the combination of these compounds to be more effective than either one alone.

Kitchen Prescription

Help from Hesperetin! You can get hesperetin from the Sunshine State fruits—oranges, grapefruit, and lemons.

Lignans. Lignans are antioxidant phytoestrogens that kill viruses and cancer. As the subject of numerous studies, lignans are being evaluated for their role in making better and safer anticancer drugs. Some lignans have shown *selective cytotoxicity*, which means they recognize and kill only cancer cells.

Dr. Lilian Thompson at the University of Toronto has conducted many studies on the effects of lignan-rich flaxseed on cancer. Flax was found to reduce the spread of skin cancer and slow its growth rate. In test-tube studies, it was also found to reduce the spread of breast cancer by 45 percent. Other researchers have found that flaxseed inhibits the growth and development of prostate cancer in animal studies.

 Kitchen Prescription

Get the Flax! Lignans are found in high concentrations in flaxseed as well as in legumes, including peas, beans, and lentils, as well as olive oil. To get the maximum benefit of lignans, buy whole flaxseed and grind them in a coffee grinder. Sprinkle over cereal or yogurt, add to smoothies, or bake into whole-grain breads and muffins.

Carotenoid Phytonutrients

Carotenoids, a group of more than six hundred related nutrients, have received substantial attention because of both their provitamin and antioxidant roles. Researchers agree that getting the full spectrum of carotenoids is the best strategy to reduce the risk of cancer; as with all compounds in foods, they work best together. Most carotenoids are yellow, orange, and red. Let's take a look at the specific carotenoid phytonutrients.

Alpha-Carotene. Alpha-carotene has gained attention as one of the carotenoid cancer crushers. Researchers at Harvard report that nonsmokers who ate the most alpha-carotene–rich foods reduced their risk of lung cancer by 63 percent. Similarly, alpha-carotene, as part of a mix of carotenoids, was found to have an inverse association with breast cancer, specifically invasive cancers that spread to the lymph nodes. Prostate cancer risk was also found to decline for men consuming alpha-carotene along with the other carotenoids.

A recent study conducted at the University of North Carolina at Chapel Hill, called the Polyp Prevention Trial, studied colon polyp recurrence and the impact of carotenoids. The study found that alpha-carotene, as part of the carotenoid arsenal, may protect against colon polyp recurrence in people who do not smoke or drink alcohol. Colon polyps increase the risk for colon cancer, so primary and secondary prevention of these growths can help reduce cancer risk and recurrence.

 Kitchen Prescription

Fourteen-Carrot Protection! Alpha-carotene can be found in carrots, carrot juice, pumpkins, and winter squash. Because it is a fat-soluble compound, you can get the most protection by cooking these foods and adding a little oil. This helps make the phytonutrients more available to your body so more gets into your bloodstream to fend off cancer.

Beta-Carotene. This antioxidant compound, which is the most well-known of the carotenoids, appears to reduce the risk for cancer in whole-food form. It is especially important to emphasize the importance of whole foods instead of dietary supplements, especially with beta-carotene. When isolated and used as a supplement, beta-carotene has been shown to increase the risk for certain cancers, including lung cancer.

 Kitchen Prescription

Get It Whole! Get your beta-carotene in sweet potatoes, carrots, cantaloupe, squash, apricots, pumpkins, and mangoes. Add heat and a little oil for optimum benefits.

Beta-Cryptoxanthin. A recent study using beta-cryptoxanthin from mandarin oranges showed that this phytonutrient reduced the number of colon cancer cells and caused apoptosis, or cell suicide, in the lab. Along with its other carotenoid cousins (including lycopene, alpha-carotene, beta-carotene, lutein, and zeaxanthin), beta-cryptoxanthin was found to be an effective agent against prostate cancer.

 Kitchen Prescription

Beat Cancer with Beta-Cryptoxanthin! You can get this compound in citrus fruits (like mandarin oranges) and sweet red peppers.

Lycopene. Lycopene is well-known for its ability to protect the heart, but it has also been noted for its prostate-protecting action. A Harvard review of seventy-two studies showed that eating tomatoes and tomato-based products significantly cuts the risk of prostate, lung, stomach, pancreatic, esophageal, breast, and cervical cancers.

 Kitchen Prescription

Love Your Lycopene! In addition to tomatoes, you can find lycopene in watermelon, guava, papaya, apricots, pink grapefruit, and blood oranges. It's fat soluble too, so cook those tomatoes well, add some extra-virgin olive oil, and toss with your favorite pasta.

Lutein and Zeaxanthin. These antioxidant carotenoids are most famous for their role in reducing the risk of age-related macular degeneration. Recent research suggests that this pair, as part of the cancer-fighting carotenoid bunch, may help to reduce the risk of certain cancers, including those of the breast and lung.

Kitchen Prescription

Go Green! Get lutein and zeaxanthin in broccoli, kale, spinach, and egg yolks.

Organosulfur Compounds

These potent cancer fighters come mainly from the mustard (Cruciferae) family of vegetables and create a distinct smell during cooking.

Isothiocyanates. Isothiocyanates are some of the most potent cancer crushers discovered. In fact, they have the ability to stop cancer that has been experimentally induced in lab studies. Isothiocyanates block the ability of carcinogens to cause cancer by calling on the body's detoxifying system (glutathione and other peptides) and making cancer cells commit suicide. Results have consistently shown that isothiocyanates, as well as other phytonutrients from the mustard family, can stop cancer at its onset and in its growth and development.

 Kitchen Prescription

Cancer-Crushing Cruciferous Veggies! You can find isothiocyanates in cruciferous vegetables, including broccoli, cauliflower, cabbage, kale, watercress, collards, and radishes.

Indoles. Indoles are also powerful anticancer compounds that help to protect against breast, colon, and other cancers. In addition, they turn off specific estrogen hormones that may encourage tumor growth.

Kitchen Prescription

Indulge in Indoles! Get your dose of indoles with broccoli, cauliflower, cabbage, kale, watercress, collards, and radishes.

Allylic Sulfur Compounds

Derived mainly from the onion (*Liliaceae*) family, these phytonutrients give the characteristic bite to onions, garlic, and other relatives of this bulb group.

Ajoene is found in garlic and is known for its blood-thinning and cholesterol-lowering properties. Applied to the skin, ajoene was found to improve basal cell carcinoma, and it has also been found to stop the development of leukemia cells by encouraging apoptosis. But the benefits don't stop there. This phytonutrient also enhances the ability of two cancer drugs, cytarabine and fludarabine, to kill cancer cells.

Allicin is a compound formed in garlic when an intact clove is crushed. An odorless amino acid, alliin, is enzymatically converted by allinase into allicin when the cloves are crushed. Allicin is thought to be one of the most biologically active compounds in garlic and has recently been found to boost the immune system, block tumor formation, and cause apoptosis in the lab.

Sulfides are also found in garlic, as well as in cabbage, broccoli, brussels sprouts, and other members of the mustard family. Diallyl disulfide (DADS), a substance that is formed from the compounds present in garlic, is known to increase levels of detoxifying enzymes in the body, including glutathione. It has also been found to inhibit the transformation of normal skin cells into cancerous ones. Several forms of sulfides, including diallyl sulfide (DAS), DADS, and diallyl trisulfide (DATS) were found to kill liver cancer cells in laboratory studies.

Kitchen Prescription

Cloves of Protection! Don't let anyone tell you garlic breath isn't beautiful. Crush garlic and mix it in with a simple dressing of extra-virgin olive oil and balsamic vinegar, and drizzle it over a big mixed green salad full of phytonutrients. Or you can enjoy it in our recipe for Garlicky Bruschetta.

Garlicky Bruschetta
4 tomatoes, chopped
4 garlic cloves, crushed
$1/_2$ shallot, diced
$1/_2$ cup fresh basil, chopped
$1/_4$ cup extra-virgin olive oil
8 slices whole-grain Italian bread, sliced

Mix all diabetes-crushing ingredients together (except bread). Let stand for 10 minutes. Toast whole-grain bread and top with tomato mixture for a dose of ajoene, allicin, sulfides, and lycopene.
Serves 8 (serving size: 1 slice bread with $1/_4$ cup tomato mixture)

Now that you have heard about how certain foods that contain fats, carbs, antioxidants, and phytonutrients can provide nutritional therapy and protection, let's move on to the next chapter, which has a whole list of foods to incorporate all of these elements into your daily diet for maximizing treatment and recovery and preventing recurrence.

Cancer-Fighting Foods

MANY PEOPLE THINK that taking supplements reaps the same benefits as proper eating. They say, "I'm getting all the same nutrients, right?" Wrong! Each fruit, vegetable, legume, or grain—like a team player or a note in a symphony—adds a nutritional element valuable to your health. Because we have only just begun exploring foods, we may be eliminating other cancer-protective elements when we rely on supplements.

Now that we've learned about the spectrum of cancer-fighting nutrients, fats, and carbohydrates, let's look at the individual foods that work together in synergy to protect against cancer and aid in treatment and recovery.

Food Synergy: The Key to Nutritional Healing

With technological advancements, scientists have isolated and identified thousands of unique phytonutrients in hundreds of different types of plant sources. Researchers are now learning that by combining these foods, the bioactive compounds work together, or synergistically, to increase health benefits. For example, when oranges, apples, grapes, and blueberries were tested both alone and together, the antioxidant activity was five times lower for the individual fruits than the combined fruit salad.

Although certain groups of fruits and vegetables have been found to be especially protective against a particular cancer, research has pointed to the conclusion that cancer prevention is best achieved by food synergy: a consumption of a wide variety of fruits and vegetables.

The thousands of phytonutrients present in whole foods behave and interact with our cells, organs, and tissues in different ways to protect our health. Although dietary supplements may contain antioxidant compounds, science shows that the balanced, natural combination of phytonutrients present in fruits and vegetables cannot be mimicked. The health benefits from eating a wide variety of these foods doesn't just apply to reducing the risk of many cancers. It also reduces the risk of other chronic diseases such as cardiovascular disease, cataracts, age-related macular degeneration, central neurodegenerative diseases, and diabetes. We examine food families and their unique cancer-fighting properties more closely in Table 5.1.

TABLE 5.1 Foods and Their Cancer-Fighting Properties

Family	Foods	Phytonutrients
Cruciferae (mustard or crucifer) family	Broccoli, brussels sprouts, cabbage, cauliflower, collard greens, kale, mustard greens, radishes, watercress	Isothiocyanates, indoles, nitriles, sulforaphane, chlorophyll
Cucurbitaceae (melon and squash) family	Cucumbers, squash (pumpkin, zucchini), cantaloupe, honeydew melon	Carotenoids, beta-carotene, alpha-carotene, beta-cryptoxanthin, zeaxanthin, lutein
Labiatae (mint) family	Basil, mint, oregano, sage, rosemary, thyme	Terpenoids, menthol, chlorophyll

TABLE 5.1 *continued*

Family	Foods	Phytonutrients
Leguminosae (bean) family	Alfalfa sprouts, beans, peas, soybeans	Phytoestrogens, lignans, protease inhibitors, isoflavones, saponins
Liliaceae (lily) family	Asparagus, chives, garlic, leeks, onions, shallots	Sulfur compounds, sulfides, allicin, diallyl sulfide
Rutacea (citrus) family	Grapefruit, lemons, limes, oranges, tangerines	Limonene, carotenoids, lycopene (blood oranges and pink grapefruit), vitamin C
Solanaceae (nightshade) family	Eggplant, peppers, potatoes, tomatoes	Lycopene, carotenoids, terpenes
Umbelliferae (carrot) family	Anise, caraway, carrots, celeriac, celery, chervil, cilantro, coriander, cumin, dill, fennel, parsley, parsnips	Carotenoids, beta-carotene, alpha-carotene, beta-cryptoxanthin, zeaxanthin, lutein, chlorophyll
Zingiberaceae (ginger) family	Ginger, turmeric	Curcumin, gingerols, zingibain
Theaceae (tea) Family	Green tea, black tea, oolong tea, white tea varieties	Catechins, polyphenols, epigallocatechin gallate (EGCG), theaflavins

Color-Coded Cuisine: Rules for Eating

Phytonutrients are natural compounds found in plant-based foods that give plants their rich pigment as well as their distinctive taste and smell. They are essentially the plant's immune system and offer protection to humans as well. There are thousands of phytonutrients that might help prevent cancer as well as provide other health benefits. They protect DNA from cancer-causing agents, promote protective enzymes, help the liver detoxify, and change estrogen to a form that is less cancer-promoting.

Dr. David Heber, Ph.D., of the UCLA Center for Human Nutrition in Los Angeles, introduced a concept that groups foods by color to simplify eating for optimum health and disease prevention. It is not necessary to know the names of the thousands of phytonutrients present in foods to reap their health benefits. In fact, choosing a variety of foods from all of the families we describe here offers the complete spectrum of nutrients needed to help protect you from developing cancer, enhance your body's response to treatment, and prevent recurrence.

The same phytonutrients that keep your cells healthy also give fruits and vegetables their colors and indicate their unique physiological roles. By color-coding your cuisine, you can translate the science of phytonutrient nutrition into delicious dishes.

❖ **Blue and purple.** These fruits and vegetables contain varying amounts of health-promoting phytonutrients such as anthocyanins and phenolics. You might remember the discussion of these phytonutrients from Chapter 4.

❖ **Green.** These vegetables contain varying amounts of phytonutrients such as lutein and indoles. Green foods are especially important in cancer prevention.

❖ **White.** White, tan, and brown fruits and vegetables contain varying amounts of phytonutrients of interest to scientists. These include ajoene, sulfides, and allicin, as well as the mineral selenium. Don't let the pale color of these foods trick you into thinking they're nutritional weaklings. Garlic and onions pack a powerful cancer-crushing punch.

✦ **Yellow and orange.** These fruits and vegetables contain varying amounts of antioxidants (such as vitamin C), as well as carotenoids (like beta-cryptoxanthin and alpha-carotene) and flavonoids. Researchers used a variety of carotenoids in the laboratory to create a "carotenoid cocktail" and determine its effects against cancer. Not ironically, these foods with a sunny disposition were found to be effective against several hormone-dependent cancers.

✦ **Red.** Specific phytonutrients in the red group, such as lycopene and anthocyanins, are being studied for their health-promoting properties. Probably the most well-researched phytonutrient, lycopene is known to protect against more than six cancers.

A to Z Foods: Your Cancer-Fighting Arsenal

Let the grocery store be your pharmacy and fill your cart with these foods to repair your cells, enhance your immune system, improve the effectiveness of your treatment, and cope with side effects. In this section, we take the color system one step further and discover the individual foods in the cancer-fighting team. We'll also show you what to look for when selecting foods, how to store them for optimum flavor and nutritional benefits, and which recipes in Chapter 9 will help you start incorporating these foods into your diet.

Apples

Grown in temperate zones throughout the world and cultivated for at least three thousand years, apple varieties now number well into the thousands. The apple has been called the "king of fruits"—and for good reason. It contains cancer crushers like phenols and quercetin, plus a soluble fiber called pectin, which helps to balance blood sugar.

❖ **Serving.** One apple (5 ounces) with skin contains 81 calories, 0.3 gram protein, 22 grams carbohydrates, no fat, no cholesterol, and 5 grams dietary fiber. The same serving provides 13 percent of the recommended daily allowance (RDA) of vitamin C (4.8 mg) and 8 percent of the RDA of vitamin E (0.8 mg).

❖ **Selecting and storing.** Available year-round, apples' peak season is from September through November when they're newly harvested. Buy firm, well-colored apples with a fresh (never musty) fragrance. The skin should be smooth and free of bruises and gouges. Store apples in a cool, dark place. They do well when placed in a plastic bag and stored in the refrigerator.

 Kitchen Prescription

Wash apples well and eat the peel to avoid losing large amounts (about 4 mg) of quercetin and fiber.

Apricots

Born in China some four thousand years ago, apricots are widely consumed by the long-living Hunza people. This cousin of the peach arrived in California with the Spanish in the eighteenth century. The orange flesh of these small wonders gives us a big clue that they're chock-full of cancer-fighting carotenoids—the group that includes alpha-carotene, beta-carotene, beta-cryptoxanthin, and others. Because this group of phytonutrients is fat soluble, enjoy your apricots with a healthy source of fat, such as nuts.

❖ **Serving.** Three apricots (4 ounces) contain 51 calories, 1.5 grams protein, 11.8 grams carbohydrates, 0.5 gram fat, no cholesterol, and 2 grams dietary fiber. The same serving provides 28 percent of the RDA of vitamin A (200 RE), 14 percent of the RDA of vitamin C (10.5 mg), 2 percent of the RDA of iron (0.4 mg), and 272 milligrams potassium.

❖ **Selecting and storing.** Because they're highly perishable and seasonal, 90 percent of fresh apricots are marketed in June and July. When buying apricots, select plump, reasonably firm fruit with a uniform color. Store in a plastic bag in the refrigerator for up to three to five days. Depending on size, you'll get eight to twelve apricots per pound.

 Kitchen Prescription

Use apricots in our yummy Tummy-Soothing Smoothie recipe, paired with ginger, or in our Fig and Apricot Compote recipe.

Artichokes

Vegetable flowers that are picked and eaten before they turn into "real" flowers, artichokes are a European staple with more than forty varieties in existence. These green globes help to fight cancer with their hefty dose of folate, which helps to ensure proper cell division, thus reducing those mutations that can lead to cancer.

❖ **Serving.** One artichoke (4.2 ounces), boiled, contains 60 calories, 4.2 grams protein, 13.4 grams carbohydrates, 0.2 gram fat, no cholesterol, and 6.5 grams dietary fiber. The same serving provides 15 percent of the RDA of folate (61.2 mcg), 16 percent of the RDA of vitamin C (12 mg), 12 percent of the RDA of magnesium (47 mg), and 316 milligrams potassium.

❖ **Selecting and storing.** Globe artichokes are available year-round, with the peak season running from March through May. Buy deep green, heavy-for-their-size artichokes with a tight leaf formation. The leaves should "squeak" when pressed together. Heavy browning on an artichoke usually indicates that it's beyond its prime. Store unwashed artichokes in a plastic bag in the refrigerator for up to four days; wash them just before cooking. Artichoke hearts are available frozen and canned, and artichoke bottoms are available canned.

 Kitchen Prescription

Try our Shells Stuffed with Ricotta, Spinach, and Artichokes recipe.

Asparagus

A member of the lily (Liliaceae) family, the edible part of asparagus is actually the young underground sprout or shoot. These spears of protection offer a good amount of folate and vitamin C, as well as the detoxifying enzyme glutathione, which is made by your liver to reduce free radical damage.

❖ **Serving.** One-half cup of raw asparagus contains 15 calories, 1.5 grams protein, 2.5 grams carbohydrates, 0.1 gram fat, no cholesterol, and 1.3 grams dietary fiber. The same serving provides 6 percent of the RDA of vitamin A (60 RE), 48 percent of the RDA of folate (95 mcg), 37 percent of the RDA of vitamin C (22.1 mg), 5 percent of the RDA of vitamin B_6 (0.1 mg), 3 percent of the RDA of iron (0.4 mg), and 218 milligrams potassium.

❖ **Selecting and storing.** The optimum season for fresh asparagus lasts from February through June, although hothouse asparagus is available year-round in some regions. It's best cooked the same day it's purchased but will keep, tightly wrapped in a plastic bag, three to four days in the refrigerator. It can also be stored standing upright in about an inch of water with a plastic bag covering the container.

 Kitchen Prescription

What's That Smell? Don't be alarmed if you notice a distinct odor. An amino acid in asparagus called asparagine causes unusual smelling urine in some people.

Avocados

Native to the tropics and subtropics, avocados are a unique fruit and concentrated source of nutrients. The California avocado has a smooth skin, while the Florida avocado ("alligator pear") has a tough and wrinkled exterior. These delicious fruits deliver 15 percent of the RDA of cancer-fighting folate per serving, plus monounsaturated fats to balance blood sugar and glutathione to neutralize free radicals. A UCLA study showed that avocados stop the growth of prostate cancer cells (as discussed in Chapter 3).

❖ **Serving.** One avocado (6 ounces) contains 204 calories, 3.8 grams protein, 13.3 grams carbohydrates, 17 grams fat, no cholesterol, and 9.3 grams dietary fiber. The same serving provides 15 percent of the RDA of folate (60 mcg), 8 percent of the RDA of vitamin B_6 (0.13 mg), 40 percent of the RDA of vitamin C (24 mg), 30 percent of the RDA of niacin (5.9 mg), 27 percent of the RDA of thiamin (0.4 mg), 26 percent of the RDA of magnesium (104 mg), 22 percent of the RDA of riboflavin (0.4 mg), 19 percent of the RDA of vitamin A (186 RE), 11 percent of the RDA of iron (1.6 mg), and 1,484 milligrams potassium.

❖ **Selecting and storing.** Like many fruits, avocados ripen best off the tree. Ripe avocados yield to gentle palm pressure, but firm, unripe fruit are what you'll usually find in the market. Select those that are unblemished and heavy for their size. To speed the ripening process, place several avocados in a paper bag and set aside at room temperature for two to four days. Ripe avocados can be stored in the refrigerator for several days. Once avocado flesh is cut and exposed to the air, it tends to discolor rapidly, so add lemon or lime juice to help prevent discoloration.

 Kitchen Prescription

A good source of healthy fat and calories and packed with other nutrients, avocados are a good choice when trying to gain back weight after cancer treatment.

Barley

Beige and shaped like a flattened oval, this grain is usually sold pearled (hulled and polished to cook more quickly). Barley can also be found in quick-cooking, whole hulled, Job's tears (large hulled grains), grits, flakes, and flour varieties. Used to make beer, whiskey, and cattle feed, barley is a gluten grain and so should be avoided by those with gluten sensitivity.

❖ **Serving.** One-half cup of cooked pearled barley contains 97 calories, 1.8 grams protein, 22.3 grams carbohydrates, 0.4 gram fat, no cholesterol, and 4.4 grams dietary fiber. The same serving provides 6 percent of the RDA of folate (12.6 mcg), 8 percent of the RDA of niacin (1.6 mg), and 7 percent of the RDA of iron (1.1 mg).

❖ **Selecting and storing.** Hulled (also called whole-grain) barley has only the outer husk removed and is the most nutritious form of the grain. Scotch barley is husked and coarsely ground. Barley grits are hulled barley grains that have been cracked into medium-coarse pieces. Hulled and Scotch barley and barley grits are generally found in health-food stores. Pearl barley has also had the bran removed and has been steamed and polished. It comes in three sizes—coarse, medium, and fine—and is good in soups and stews.

Kitchen Prescription

Barley also contains tocotrienol, a form of vitamin E, and selenium, a mineral that is part of antioxidant enzymes and seems to have a special role in protecting against prostate cancer.

Beans

Part of the Leguminosae family, a good protein source, and a food with a low glycemic index, beans should take a starring role at the dinner table for anyone who wants to prevent cancer. Packed inside you'll find isoflavones, lignans, and folate, each of which may play a unique role in preventing cancer. (Refer back to Chapter 4.)

✦ **Serving.** One-half cup of cooked black beans contains 113 calories, 7.6 grams protein, 20.4 grams carbohydrates, 0.4 gram fat, no cholesterol, and 7.5 grams dietary fiber. The same serving size provides 32 percent of the RDA of folate (64.2 mcg), 13 percent of the RDA of magnesium (51.6 mg), and 270.2 milligrams potassium.

✦ **Selecting and storing.** Dried beans must usually be soaked in water for several hours or overnight to rehydrate them before cooking. Beans labeled "quick-cooking" have been presoaked and redried before packaging. They require no presoaking and take considerably less time to prepare. The texture of these quick beans, however, is not as firm to the bite as regular dried beans. Store dried beans in an airtight container for up to a year.

 Kitchen Prescription

The following recipes are five quick ways to incorporate beans:

* Rice, Corn, and Bean Medley with Cilantro, Coriander, and Cumin
* Black Bean and Vegetable Wraps
* Eggplant, Spinach, and Garbanzo Bean Curry
* Southwestern Bean Salad
* Minestrone

Beets

Root vegetables that were taken to Europe and the British Isles by Roman soldiers, beets can be boiled or used raw in juices. Beeturia can create red-colored urine caused by the pigment in beets, so don't panic if this happens. Beets are rich in anthocyanins and beta-cryptoxanthin.

* **Serving.** One-half cup of cooked, sliced beets contains 26 calories, 0.9 gram protein, 5.7 grams carbohydrates, no fat, no cholesterol, and 1.4 grams dietary fiber. The same serving provides 23 percent of the RDA of folate (45.2 mcg), 8 percent of the RDA of vitamin C (4.7 mg), 8 percent of the RDA of magnesium (31 mg), 3 percent of the RDA of iron (0.5 mg), and 265 milligrams potassium.

* **Selecting and storing.** Beets are available year-round and should be chosen by their firmness and smooth skins. Small or medium beets are generally more tender than large ones. If the

beet greens are attached, they should be crisp and bright. Because they leach moisture from the bulb, greens should be removed as soon as you get them home. Leave about one inch of the stem attached to prevent loss of nutrients and color during cooking. Store beets in a plastic bag in the refrigerator for up to three weeks. Just before cooking, wash beets gently so as not to pierce the thin skin, which could cause nutrient and color loss. Peel beets after they've been cooked.

 Kitchen Prescription

Wash the beets well, use a juicer, and mix with spinach and carrot juices for a nutrient-packed drink.

Blueberries

These berries have been enjoyed by Native Americans and Pilgrims and are one of the best-known sources of antioxidants. Blueberries provide a delicious dose of vitamin C (a whopping 315 percent of the RDA for a cup), plus anthocyanins.

✤ **Serving.** One cup of blueberries contains 82 calories, 1 gram protein, 20.5 grams carbohydrates, 0.6 gram fat, no cholesterol, and 3.5 grams dietary fiber. The same serving provides 315 percent of the RDA of vitamin C (189 mg) and 129 milligrams potassium.

✤ **Selecting and storing.** Choose blueberries that are firm, uniform in size, and indigo blue with a silvery frost. Discard shriveled or moldy berries. Do not wash them until you're ready to use them, and store them (preferably in a single layer) in a moisture-proof container in the refrigerator for up to five days.

Kitchen Prescription

Try our Blueberry Mango Soy Smoothie or sip on our Banana Berry
Cooler.

Broccoli

A descendant of cabbage, broccoli is a member of the cancer-
fighting cruciferous (mustard) family of vegetables. Although
most broccoli is green, in times past, purple, red, cream, and
brown varieties were popular. These trees to ease disease contain
indoles, sulforaphane, lutein, and quercetin. (Learn more about
how each of these compounds fights cancer in Chapter 4.)

✤ **Serving.** One-half cup of cooked broccoli contains 23 calories, 2.3 grams protein, 6 grams carbohydrates, 0.2 gram fat, no
cholesterol, and 2.6 grams dietary fiber. The same serving provides 11 percent of the RDA of vitamin A (110 RE), 27 percent
of the RDA of folate (53.3 mcg), 82 percent of the RDA of vitamin C (49 mg), 10 percent of the RDA of vitamin B_6 (0.2 mg),
6 percent of the RDA of iron (0.9 mg), and 127 milligrams
potassium.

✤ **Selecting and storing.** Look for broccoli with a deep, strong
color—green or green with purple. The buds should be tightly
closed and the leaves crisp. Refrigerate it unwashed, in an airtight
bag, for up to four days.

> **Kitchen Prescription**
>
> Find broccoli in our recipes for Triple Crucifer Soup, Shrimp and Broccolini Stir-Fry, and Shiitake-and-Rappini-Stuffed Chicken Breasts. What is rappini? Also called broccoli rabe, it has six- to nine-inch stalks and scattered clusters of tiny broccoli-like buds. It's also called brocoletti di rape, rape, and rapini. The greens have a pungent and bitter flavor, but are tasty when sautéed in olive oil with garlic.

Brussels Sprouts

These members of the crucifer (mustard) family are vegetable flowers that are picked and eaten before they progress into a "real" flower. Developed in Belgium several hundred years ago and named for the country's capital, these vegetables are offshoots of cabbage. Indoles and sulforaphane are found in brussels sprouts. One of the indole compounds, indole-3-carbinol (IC3), may be helpful for inhibiting breast and prostate cancer.

❖ **Serving.** One-half cup of boiled brussels sprouts contains 30 calories, 2 grams protein, 6.8 grams carbohydrates, 0.4 gram fat, no cholesterol, and 3.4 grams dietary fiber. The same serving provides 23 percent of the RDA of folate (46.8 mcg), 81 percent of the RDA of vitamin C (48.4 mg), 6 percent of the RDA of iron (0.9 mg), and 247.3 milligrams potassium.

❖ **Selecting and storing.** Buy small, bright green sprouts with compact heads. Store unwashed sprouts in an airtight plastic bag in the refrigerator for up to three days.

Kitchen Prescription

Use some lemon juice to complement the distinct flavor of these infamous veggies. Caraway is also a nice complement.

Buckwheat

A triangular seed from a fruit relative of rhubarb and sorrel, buckwheat has a nutty flavor and is sold roasted (kasha); whole grain cracked; or as unroasted groats, grits, or flour. Buckwheat is rich in flavonoids, those defense mechanisms in plants that also fend off cancer. It is also a gluten-free grain.

✤ **Serving.** One-half cup of buckwheat groats (cooked) contains 77 calories, 2.8 grams protein, 16.75 grams carbohydrates, 0.5 gram fat, no cholesterol, and 2.7 grams dietary fiber. The same serving provides 7 percent of the RDA of folate (13.9 mcg), 13 percent of the RDA of magnesium (43 mg), and 5 percent of the RDA of iron (0.8 mg).

✤ **Selecting and storing.** Buckwheat groats are the hulled, crushed kernels, which are usually cooked in a manner similar to rice. Groats come in coarse, medium, and fine grinds. Kasha, which is roasted buckwheat groats, has a toastier, nuttier flavor. All varieties can be stored in an airtight container in a cool, dry place.

Kitchen Prescription

One flavonoid found in buckwheat is quercetin. As an antioxidant, it combats the destructive free radical molecules that play a part in many diseases. Try it in our Pumpkin Buckwheat Flapjacks.

Bulgur

Simple wheat kernels that have been steamed, dried, and cracked, this grain is often not cooked at all, but soaked until tender. Bulgur can be found in fine, medium, and coarse granulations.

✤ **Serving.** One-half cup of cooked bulgur contains 76 calories, 2.8 grams of protein, 17 grams of carbohydrates, 0.2 gram fat, no cholesterol, and 4.1 grams of dietary fiber.

✤ **Selecting and storing.** Bulgur has a tender, chewy texture. Store it in a cool, dry place at room temperature.

Kitchen Prescription

Full of fiber and ferulic acid, try our Tabbouleh Primavera recipe to include bulgur in your diet. Tabbouleh is also offered at the grocery store in the deli section if you're pressed for time.

Cabbage

A member of the cancer-fighting crucifer (mustard) family of vegetables, cabbage comes in numerous varieties, including red cabbage, green cabbage, napa cabbage, savoy cabbage, and bok choy. Isothiocyanates, indoles, dithiolthiones, and phenols team up to decrease the hormones that encourage tumor growth and enhance the body's production of detoxifying enzymes. When you choose purple cabbage, you'll also get a dose of anthocyanins. Sauerkraut, a fermented cabbage, is especially high in these protective compounds and also contains prebiotics that benefit the digestive system.

✤ **Serving.** One-half cup of cooked, shredded green cabbage contains 16 calories, 0.7 gram protein, 3.6 grams carbohydrates, 0.2 gram fat, no cholesterol, and 1.8 grams dietary fiber. The same serving provides 8 percent of the RDA of folate (15.2 mcg) and 30 percent of the RDA of vitamin C (18.2 mg).

✤ **Selecting and storing.** Choose a cabbage with fresh, crisp-looking leaves that are firmly packed—the head should be heavy for its size. Cabbage may be refrigerated, tightly wrapped, for about a week.

 Kitchen Prescription

In the Raw! Boiling cabbage removes about half of its indoles. Try fresh cabbage sliced thin and tossed into green salads for a sweet crunch and cancer-fighting punch. Try our Triple Crucifer Soup or Crisp Asian Salad recipes to increase your cabbage intake.

Canola Oil

Derived from canola seed and produced in Canada, this oil contains the lowest level of saturated fat of any oil.

✤ **Serving.** One tablespoon contains 124 calories, no protein, no carbohydrates, 14 grams fat, 1 gram saturated fatty acids, 8 grams monounsaturated fat, 4.2 grams polyunsaturated fatty acids, 1.2 grams omega-3s, no cholesterol, and no dietary fiber. The same serving provides 13 percent of the RDA for vitamin E (2.9 mg).

✤ **Selecting and storing.** Store canola oil in a cool, dry place away from sunlight.

Kitchen Prescription

Canola oil provides a trio of the good fats—monounsaturated fat, omega-3 fatty acids, and omega-6 fatty acids—that protect against disease (see Chapter 3).

Cantaloupes

This orange-fleshed melon was named after the Italian town of Cantalupoa, meaning "wolf howl." Along with a whopping 186 percent of the RDA of vitamin C and 86 percent of the RDA of vitamin A, cantaloupe also adds carotenoids to the mix.

❖ **Serving.** One-half raw cantaloupe (9.5 ounces) contains 95 calories, 2.5 grams protein, 22.4 grams carbohydrates, 0.8 gram fat, no cholesterol, and 2.5 grams dietary fiber. The same serving provides 86 percent of the RDA of vitamin A (861 RE), 23 percent of the RDA of folate (45.5 mcg), 186 percent of the RDA of vitamin C (112.7 mg), 20 percent of the RDA of vitamin B_6 (0.4 mg), and 825 milligrams potassium.

❖ **Selecting and storing.** Choose cantaloupes that are heavy for their size; have a sweet, fruity fragrance and a thick, well-raised netting; and yield slightly to pressure at the blossom end. Avoid melons with soft spots or an overly strong odor. Store unripe cantaloupes at room temperature and ripe melons in the refrigerator. Cantaloupes easily absorb other food odors, so if you're refrigerating one for more than a day or two, wrap it in plastic wrap.

Kitchen Prescription

Try it in our Grilled Grouper with Cilantro Cantaloupe Salsa.

Carrots

As root vegetables that spread from the Middle East to Greece, Rome, and later Europe, the earliest carrots were not orange but multicolored. In the 1500s, the carrot showed up in Western Europe, and Dutch crossbreeders developed the modern, orange carrot over the following century. Carrots provide a bevy of nutrients to support the immune system and ally in the fight against cancer, including alpha-carotene, beta-carotene, and other carotenoids.

❖ **Serving.** One medium carrot (2.5 ounces) contains 31 calories, 0.7 gram protein, 5.6 grams carbohydrates, 0.1 gram fat, no cholesterol, and 2 grams dietary fiber. The same serving provides 202 percent of the RDA of vitamin A (2,025 RE), 5 percent of the RDA of folate (10 mcg), 11 percent of the RDA of vitamin C (6.7 mg), and 233 milligrams potassium.

❖ **Selecting and storing.** Choose carrots that are firm and smooth. Avoid those with cracks or any that have begun to soften and wither. Remove carrot greenery as soon as possible because it robs the roots of moisture and vitamins. Store carrots in a plastic bag in your refrigerator's vegetable bin. Avoid storing them near apples, which emit ethylene gas that can give carrots a bitter taste.

 Kitchen Prescription

These fat-soluble phytonutrients are better absorbed by the body when cooked (with a bit of oil), but juicing carrots is also a great way to get their benefits.

Cauliflower

A member of the crucifer (mustard) family of vegetables, the name *cauliflower* comes from the Latin *caulis* ("stalk") and *floris* ("flower"). Cauliflower comes in three basic colors: white (the most popular and readily available), green, and purple (a vibrant violet that turns pale green when cooked). Broccoflower is a hybrid of broccoli and cauliflower.

❖ **Serving.** One-half cup of cooked cauliflower contains 15 calories, 1.2 grams protein, 2.9 grams carbohydrates, 0.1 gram fat, no cholesterol, and 1 gram dietary fiber. The same serving provides 16 percent of the RDA of folate (31.7 mcg), 57 percent of the RDA of vitamin C (34.3 mg), and 200 milligrams potassium.

❖ **Selecting and storing.** Choose a firm cauliflower with compact florets; the leaves should be crisp and green with no sign of yellowing. The size of the head doesn't affect the quality. Refrigerate raw cauliflower, tightly wrapped, for three to five days; cooked, it will last for one to three days.

 Kitchen Prescription

Get the mild child of the crucifer (mustard) family in our Triple Crucifer Soup recipe for a healthy dose of cancer crushers, including glucosinolates, indoles, sulforaphane, and dithiolthiones.

Cherries

Close cousins to the plum, cherries can be sweet or sour, red or black. Rich in flavonoids and anthocyanins, enjoy them in smoothies, on top of whole-grain cereal, or straight out of the carton.

✤ **Serving.** Ten raw sweet cherries (2.4 ounces) contain 50 calories, 0.9 gram protein, 11.3 grams carbohydrates, 0.7 gram fat, no cholesterol, and 1.5 grams dietary fiber. The same serving provides 8 percent of the RDA of vitamin C (4.8 mg), 2 percent of the RDA of iron (0.3 mg), and 152 milligrams potassium.

✤ **Selecting and storing.** Most fresh cherries are available from May (June for sour cherries) through August. Choose brightly colored, shiny, plump fruit. Sweet cherries should be firm but not hard; sour varieties should be medium-firm. Store unwashed cherries in a plastic bag in the refrigerator.

 Kitchen Prescription

Put the Freeze on Disease! Cherries are one of the fruits you can find in the freezer section of your grocery store, making them both economical and ideal for tossing into a quick, icy cold, cancer-fighting smoothie.

Collards

Members of the cancer-fighting crucifer (mustard) family of vegetables, these greens are common in the Southern diet. Collards deliver a whole host of the organosulfur compounds that we talked about in Chapter 4, including glucosinolates, indoles, and sulforaphane.

✤ **Serving.** One-half cup of chopped, cooked collard greens contains 13 calories, 0.9 gram protein, 3.9 grams carbohydrates, 0.1 gram fat, no cholesterol, and 1.8 grams dietary fiber. The same serving provides 21 percent of the RDA of vitamin A (211 RE) and 16 percent of the RDA of vitamin C (9.3 mg).

✤ **Selecting and storing.** Collards' peak season is January through April, but they're available year-round in most markets.

Look for crisp green leaves with no evidence of yellowing, wilting, or insect damage. Refrigerate collard greens in a plastic bag for three to five days.

 Kitchen Prescription

Sauté collards with a little olive oil and serve with lemon juice and folate-rich black-eyed peas for a nutrient-packed Southern delight!

Cranberries

Grown in bogs throughout Asia, Europe, and North America, this fruit is best known for its ability to reduce the incidence of bladder infections. But cranberries do more than that. A potent source of ellagic acid—the compound that stops the cell mutations that can lead to cancer—and anthocyanins that defend cells against cancer-causing agents.

❖ **Serving.** One cup of raw cranberries contains 46 calories, 0.4 gram protein, 12.1 grams carbohydrates, 0.2 gram fat, no cholesterol, and 4.4 grams of dietary fiber. The same serving provides 21 percent of the RDA of vitamin C (12.8 mg).

❖ **Selecting and storing.** Harvested between Labor Day and Halloween, the peak market period for cranberries is from October through December. They're usually packaged in twelve-ounce plastic bags. Discard any berries that are discolored or shriveled. Cranberries can be refrigerated, tightly wrapped, for at least two months or frozen up to a year.

 Kitchen Prescription

Get the benefits of cranberries with our Banana Berry Cooler.

Eggplant

A flowering vegetable native to India, the many varieties of this delicious veggie range in color from rich purple to white, in length from two to twelve inches, and in shape from oblong to round. Eggplant, with its purple skin, contains anthocyanins.

❖ **Serving.** One-half cup of cooked eggplant contains 13 calories, 0.4 gram protein, 3.2 grams carbohydrates, 0.1 gram fat, no cholesterol, and 1.2 grams of dietary fiber. The same serving provides 3 percent of the RDA of folate (6.9 mcg) and 119 milligrams potassium.

❖ **Selecting and storing.** Available year-round, eggplant's peak season is August and September. Choose a firm, smooth-skinned eggplant that feels heavy for its size; avoid those with soft or brown spots. It should be stored in a cool, dry place and used within a day or two of purchase. If longer storage is necessary, place the eggplant in the refrigerator vegetable drawer.

 Kitchen Prescription

Try our Eggplant, Spinach, and Garbanzo Bean Curry or our Mediterranean Gateau for two delicious ways to get the benefits of anthocyanins.

Fish

Fish has been the subject of much research over the past twenty years since Danish researchers found a link between fish-eating Eskimos and low rates of heart disease. We now know that because they have abundant omega-3 fatty acids, protein, and bountiful B vitamins, fish have beneficial effects on cancer as well.

✤ **Serving.** A 3-ounce serving of salmon, baked or broiled, contains 149 calories, 20.5 grams protein, 0.4 gram carbohydrates, 6.8 grams fat, 35.7 milligrams cholesterol, and no dietary fiber. The same serving provides 122 percent of the RDA of niacin (24.5 mg), 115 percent of the RDA of vitamin B_{12} (2.3 mcg), and 20 percent of the RDA of phosphorus (238 mg).

✤ **Selecting and storing.** When available, choose wild over farm-raised salmon. (See Chapter 3 to get the real scoop on omega-3s and the dish on fish.)

 Kitchen Prescription

Fishing for Health! Cold-water fish such as tuna, mackerel, herring, and sardines have higher amounts of omega-3s than do their warm-water kin. In fact, a 3½-ounce portion of sardines contains 5.1 grams of omega-3s, while the same portion of chinook salmon, Atlantic mackerel, and pink salmon contains 3.0 grams, 2.2 grams, and 1.9 grams, respectively. Troll our Fish and Seafood recipe section for perfect fish dishes.

Flaxseed

An ancient culinary staple used as early as 3000 B.C. and touted by Hippocrates for its ability to relieve intestinal discomfort, flaxseed offers a one-two punch of powerful cancer fighters—omega-3 fats and lignans. In fact, this small seed is the richest known source of plant lignans found to be effective against breast and other hormone-dependent cancers.

✤ **Serving.** Two tablespoons of ground flaxseed contains 80 calories, 3.2 grams protein, no carbohydrates, 5.5 grams fat, no cholesterol, and 4.5 grams dietary fiber.

✦ **Selecting and storing.** Store flaxseed in the refrigerator or freezer, where it will keep for up to six months.

 Kitchen Prescription

The Daily Grind! Get out your coffee grinder to get the most out of these phytonutrient-packed seeds. The tough outer shell prevents many of the cancer-fighting nutrients from being absorbed, so grind away for better health!

Garlic

The medicinal star of the onion family, three major types of garlic are available in the United States: white-skinned, strongly flavored American garlic, and Mexican and Italian garlic, both of which have mauve-colored skins and a somewhat milder flavor. Elephant garlic (which is not a true garlic, but a relative of the leek) is the most mildly flavored of all. Garlic destroys more than seventy different bacteria (including encephalitis and tuberculosis) and seventeen strains of fungi.

✦ **Serving.** One ounce of garlic contains no calories, no protein, no fat, and no carbohydrates. It does contain 15 percent of the RDA for vitamin C and 15 percent of the RDA for vitamin B$_6$. Garlic contains allicin, diallyl sulfide, ajoene, and quercetin.

✦ **Selecting and storing.** Fresh garlic is available year-round. Purchase firm, plump bulbs with dry skins. Avoid heads with soft or shriveled cloves and those stored in the refrigerated section of the produce department. Store fresh garlic in an open container (away from other foods) in a cool, dark place. Properly stored, unbroken bulbs can be kept up to eight weeks, although they will begin to dry out toward the end of that time. Once broken from the bulb, individual cloves will keep from three to ten days.

Kitchen Prescription

Get Out the Garlic Press! These flavorful bulbs contain allicin, diallyl sulfide, ajoene, and quercetin, each of which has a unique ability to call on the body's detoxifying enzymes and enhance the immune system.

Ginger

A member of the ginger (Zingiberaceae) family, which also includes turmeric, most ginger comes from Jamaica, India, Africa, and China. Although not as potent as turmeric, ginger contains some compounds, including gingerols, that help to reduce nausea during treatment.

✢ **Serving.** One tablespoon of fresh ginger contains 4 calories, 0.1 gram protein, 0.9 gram carbohydrates, 0.1 gram fat, no cholesterol, and 0.1 gram dietary fiber. The same serving provides 46 milligrams potassium.

✢ **Selecting and storing.** Look for gingerroot with smooth skin and a fresh, spicy fragrance. Fresh, unpeeled ginger, tightly wrapped, can be refrigerated for up to three weeks and frozen for up to six months.

Kitchen Prescription

Ginger has long been revered for its ability to quell a queasy stomach and has even been found to be effective against motion sickness. If you're going through cancer treatment, you may want to try it in our Tummy-Soothing Smoothie.

Grapefruit

A member of the citrus (Rutacea) family of fruits grown in Florida, the grapefruit has long been purported as a weight-loss aid and also has a juicy role in cancer prevention. Packed with compounds like pectin, flavonoids, naringin, limonoids, lycopene (red grapefruit), and d-limonene, grapefruit is portable protection!

❖ **Serving.** One-half grapefruit contains 45 calories, 1 gram protein, 12 grams carbohydrates, 0.1 gram fat, no cholesterol, and 1.6 grams dietary fiber. The same serving provides 6 percent of the RDA of folate (11.8 mcg) and 66 percent of the RDA of vitamin C (39.3 mg).

❖ **Selecting and storing.** Fresh grapefruit is available year-round: those from Arizona and California are on the market from about January through August; and Florida and Texas grapefruits usually arrive around October and last through June. Choose fruit that have thin, fine-textured, brightly colored skin. They should be firm yet springy when held in the palm and pressed. Grapefruit keep best when wrapped in a plastic bag and placed in the vegetable drawer of the refrigerator for up to two weeks.

 Kitchen Prescription

Try this citrus fruit in our Spinach and Grapefruit Salad.

Guava

This sweet, fragrant tropical fruit grows in its native South America as well as in California, Florida, and Hawaii. There are many varieties of guavas, which can range from the size of a small egg to that of a medium apple. Not only does this tropical delight deliver 275 percent of the RDA of vitamin C, plus a good amount of vitamin B_6, but its orange flesh screams "carotenoids."

❖ **Serving.** One raw guava (2.7 ounces) contains 46 calories, 0.8 gram protein, 11.4 grams carbohydrates, 0.4 gram fat, no cholesterol, and 4.5 grams dietary fiber. The same serving provides 7 percent of the RDA of vitamin A (71 RE), 275 percent of the RDA of vitamin C (165.1 mg), 10 percent of the RDA of vitamin B_6 (0.2 mg), 6 percent of the RDA of niacin (1.1 mg), and 25.6 milligrams potassium.

❖ **Selecting and storing.** Choose fruit that give to gentle palm pressure but have not yet begun to show spots. To be eaten raw, guavas should be very ripe. Ripen green ones at room temperature. Store ripe fruit in the vegetable drawer of the refrigerator for up to four days.

 Kitchen Prescription

This delectable fruit can easily be incorporated into smoothies or served in a light salad.

Kale

A leafy green member of the cancer-fighting crucifer (mustard) family of vegetables, kale's leaves are deep green tinged with shades of blue or purple. This cousin of broccoli provides indoles, sulforaphane, and lutein.

❖ **Serving.** One-half cup of chopped, cooked kale contains 21 calories, 1.2 grams protein, 3.7 grams carbohydrates, 0.3 gram fat, no cholesterol, and 1.3 grams dietary fiber. The same serving provides 48 percent of the RDA of vitamin A (481 RE), 45 percent of the RDA of vitamin C (26.7 mg), and 4 percent of the RDA of iron (0.6 mg).

✤ **Selecting and storing.** Kale's peak season is during the winter months, although it's available year-round in most parts of the country. Choose richly colored, relatively small bunches of kale, avoiding any with limp or yellowing leaves. Store it in the coldest section of the refrigerator for no longer than two or three days.

 Kitchen Prescription

Steam or sauté kale and serve with lemon juice for a perfect side dish to accompany any meal.

Kiwi

Native to eastern Asia where several species of *Actinidia* grow wild, this fuzzy fruit is now cultivated in both New Zealand and California. It's part of the "green" family in your cancer-fighting palate.

✤ **Serving.** One kiwi (2.5 ounces) contains 46 calories, 0.8 gram protein, 11.3 grams carbohydrates, 0.3 gram fat, no cholesterol, and 2.6 grams dietary fiber. The same serving provides 1 percent of the RDA of vitamin A (13 RE), 124 percent of the RDA of vitamin C (74.5 mg), 2 percent of the RDA of niacin (0.4 mg), and 252 milligrams potassium.

✤ **Selecting and storing.** Kiwi is available year-round. Choose kiwi that yields slightly to pressure. Ripe fruit can be stored in the refrigerator for up to three weeks.

Kitchen Prescription

Quick Kiwi Trick! Getting into these suckers can be tough. Here's how: cut the ends of the kiwi off, and slide a spoon between the thin brown skin and the flesh. Move the spoon in a circle and the kiwi pops out. Voilà! Also, try kiwi in our Emerald Fruit Salad.

Leeks

Members of the onion family and native to Mediterranean countries, leeks are mild in taste and have a sweet flavor. Add leeks to soups or the stockpot to add a deep flavor that cannot be achieved by onions alone. Leeks contain sulfur compounds and kaempferol.

❖ **Serving.** One-half cup boiled leeks contains 16 calories, 0.4 gram protein, 4 grams carbohydrates, 0.2 gram fat, no cholesterol, and 0.6 gram dietary fiber.

❖ **Selecting and storing.** Leeks are available year-round in most regions. Choose those with crisp, brightly colored leaves and an unblemished white portion. Avoid any with withered or yellow-spotted leaves. The smaller the leek, the more tender it will be. Refrigerate leeks in a plastic bag for up to five days. When using leeks, wash well between leaves to remove all sand and grit prior to cooking.

 Kitchen Prescription

Try leeks in our recipe for Mustard Baked Salmon with Lentils.

Lemon

Citrus fruits cultivated in tropical and temperate climates around the world, lemons add zest and an abundance of vitamin C to foods and beverages. With a sunny disposition and a tremendous pucker power, this sassy fruit provides compounds such as limonene and terpenes to keep cancer at bay.

✦ **Serving.** One tablespoon of lemon juice contains 4 calories, 0.1 gram protein, 1.4 grams carbohydrates, no fat, no cholesterol, and no fiber. The same serving provides 11 percent of the RDA of vitamin C (75 mg).

✦ **Selecting and storing.** Lemons are available year-round, peaking during the summer months. Choose fruit with smooth, brightly colored skin and no tinge of green. Lemons should be firm, plump, and heavy for their size. Depending on their condition when purchased, they can be refrigerated in a plastic bag for two to three weeks.

 Kitchen Prescription

Citrus A-Peel! Limonene, which appears in high concentrations in lemon peel, has been found to be especially potent against cancer. Steep your tea with a lemon wedge for a bite filled with phytonutrients!

Lentils

Members of the bean family, lentils come in red, green, and brown varieties. Full of folate, the B vitamin found to help reduce the risk for breast and colon cancers, they also have isoflavones that discourage cancer growth.

❖ **Serving.** One-half cup of cooked lentils contains 101 calories, 7.4 grams protein, 18.4 grams carbohydrates, no fat, no cholesterol, and 9 grams dietary fiber. The same serving provides 86 percent of the RDA of folate (172.7 mcg), 15 percent of the RDA of iron (0.8 mg), and 7 percent of the RDA of thiamin (0.1 mg).

❖ **Selecting and storing.** Dry lentils should be stored in an airtight container at room temperature and will keep up to a year. You can also choose canned lentils for a fast, no-fuss alternative.

 Kitchen Prescription

Try lentils in our Mustard Baked Salmon with Lentils recipe.

Mangoes

Cultivated in India for several thousand years, mangoes come in hundreds of varieties. This tropical fruit is high in antioxidants and can be blended into smoothies or baked into bread. Coupled with vitamins A and C, the orange-yellow color is a dead giveaway that these fibrous fruits are high in carotenoids.

❖ **Serving.** One raw mango (7.3 ounces) contains 128 calories, 1 gram protein, 33.4 grams carbohydrates, 0.6 gram fat, no cholesterol, and 3.7 grams dietary fiber. The same serving provides 77 percent of the RDA of vitamin A (766 RE), 90 percent of the RDA of vitamin C (54 mg), 24 percent of the RDA of vitamin E (2.4 mg), and 14 percent of the RDA of vitamin B_6 (0.28 mg).

❖ **Selecting and storing.** Mangoes are in season from May to September, although imported fruit is in the stores sporadically throughout the remainder of the year. Look for fruit with an unblemished, yellow skin blushed with red.

Kitchen Prescription

Try them in our Blueberry Mango Soy Smoothie.

Mushrooms

A type of edible fungus, mushrooms are consumed worldwide and often described as the "meat" of the vegetable kingdom. Different varieties of mushrooms contain various cancer-fighting compounds. Shiitake mushrooms contain lentinan, which enhances the activity of natural killer cells, and macrophages that destroy tumor cells. However, some people are allergic or sensitive to mushrooms. Individuals with intestinal yeast overgrowth, yeast sensitivities, or mold allergies may have crossover reactions to the fungi family.

❖ **Serving.** One-half cup of button mushrooms contains 21 calories, 1.7 grams protein, 4 grams carbohydrates, 0.4 gram fat, no cholesterol, and 1.7 grams dietary fiber. The same serving provides 7 percent of the RDA of folate (14.4 mcg), 18 percent of the RDA of riboflavin (0.2 mg), 7 percent of the RDA of iron (1 mg), and 278 milligrams potassium.

❖ **Selecting and storing.** Most mushrooms are available year-round but are at their peak in fall and winter. Look for those that are firm and evenly colored with tightly closed caps. If all the gills are showing, the mushrooms are past their prime. Fresh mushrooms should be placed on a tray in a single layer, covered with a damp paper towel and refrigerated for up to three days. Before use, wipe them with a damp paper towel or, if necessary, rinse them with cold water and dry thoroughly.

Kitchen Prescription

Fabulous Fungus! Mushrooms are a versatile food, taking on the flavors of the herbs, spices, oils, and other foods you pair them with. Try our Herbed Polenta with Grilled Portobello Mushrooms for a Tuscan flair to this fabulous fungus.

Nuts

Scientists speculate that nuts may have been around tens of millions of years ago when the continents were still fused in a landmass known as Pangaea. We know this because nuts are native to both the Old World and the New World. Cultivated for twelve thousand years, they are one of nature's richest foods. More than three hundred types of nuts exist, but those most commonly enjoyed include almonds, Brazil nuts, cashews, chestnuts, coconuts, hazelnuts, peanuts, pecans, pistachios, walnuts, hickory nuts, pine nuts, and macadamia nuts.

✤ **Serving.** See the packaging of individual nuts for nutritional information.

✤ **Selecting and storing.** Store nuts in closed containers in the refrigerator or freezer to avoid rancidity. It is best to buy fresh raw nuts in the shell, as they will store longer than shelled, cooked varieties.

Kitchen Prescription

Loaded with the good fats and minerals, nuts are a great snack and are easily incorporated into salads and smoothies. One of the most healthful choice is raw, unblanched almonds.

Oats

A highly rich protein grain eaten in prepared cereals or alone as a hot cereal, oats are an American staple. They provide tocotrienol (a natural form of vitamin E), selenium, beta-glucan, and phytates that team up to boost immunity.

✤ **Serving.** One cup of cooked oatmeal (½ cup dry) contains 150 calories, 5.5 grams protein, 27 grams carbohydrates, 3 grams fat, no cholesterol, and 4 grams dietary fiber. The same serving size provides 13 percent of the RDA for thiamin (0.2 mg), 31 percent of the RDA for magnesium (107 mg), and 9 percent of the RDA for iron (1.9 mg).

✤ **Selecting and storing.** Store oats in a cool, dry place.

 Kitchen Prescription

One of Mom's old remedies for upset stomachs and general malaise, oatmeal can be a comfort food during cancer treatment.

Olive Oil

Made by pressing tree-ripened olives to extract a flavorful, monounsaturated oil that is prized throughout the world for both cooking and salad dressings, most olive oils come from California or are imported from France, Greece, Italy, and Spain. The flavor, color, and fragrance of olive oils can vary depending on distinctions such as growing region and the crop's condition. Olive oil contains monounsaturated fats and phenols that may be effective against breast cancer.

❖ **Serving.** One tablespoon of extra-virgin olive oil contains 120 calories, no protein, no carbohydrates, 14 grams fat, no cholesterol, and no dietary fiber.

❖ **Selecting and storing.** Olive oil should be stored in a cool, dark place for up to six months. It can also be refrigerated, in which case it will last up to a year.

 Kitchen Prescription

All olive oils are graded according to the degree of acidity they contain. The best are cold-pressed, a chemical-free process that involves only pressure, which produces a naturally low level of acidity. Extra-virgin olive oil, the result of the first cold-pressing of the olives, is only 1 percent acid. It is considered the finest and fruitiest of the olive oils and is therefore also the most expensive. It can range from a champagne color to greenish-golden to bright green. In general, the deeper the color, the more intense the olive flavor and the more phytonutrients are present.

Onions

Members of the lily family, onions have two main classifications: green onions and dry onions (which are simply mature onions with a juicy flesh covered with dry, papery skin). With their quercetin, sulfur compounds, and anthocyanins (in red and purple onions), these bulbs are bursting with cancer-fighting allies.

❖ **Serving.** One medium, raw onion contains 60 calories, 2 grams protein, 14 grams carbohydrates, no fat, no cholesterol, and 3 grams dietary fiber. The same serving provides 18 percent of the RDA of vitamin C (12 mg).

❖ **Selecting and storing.** When buying onions, choose those that are heavy for their size with dry, papery skins and no signs of spotting or moistness. Avoid onions with soft spots. Look for green onions that are bright white on the bottom, with smooth green tops and no sign of browning. Store them in a cool, dry place with good air circulation for up to two months (depending on their condition when purchased). Once cut, an onion should be tightly wrapped, refrigerated, and used within four days.

 Kitchen Prescription

Toss onions into salads, dice and sauté them for sauces, or chop and add them to soups.

Oranges

The most popular citrus fruit, oranges are believed to have originated in southeast Asia and been brought to the New World by Columbus. Along with vitamins C and A, oranges provide a spectrum of flavonoids, including hesperetin, pectin, and glutathione.

✤ **Serving.** One orange (approximately 4.6 ounces) contains 62 calories, 1.3 grams protein, 15.4 grams carbohydrates, 0.2 gram fat, no cholesterol, and 3 grams dietary fiber. The same serving provides 20 percent of the RDA of folate (39.7 mcg), 92 percent of the RDA of vitamin C (69.7 mg), 13 percent of the RDA of thiamin (0.2 mg), 4 percent of the RDA of calcium (52 mg), and 237 milligrams potassium.

✤ **Selecting and storing.** Fresh oranges are available year-round at different times, depending on the variety. Choose fruit that is firm and heavy for its size, with no mold or spongy spots. Oranges can be stored at (cool) room temperature for a day or so, but they should then be put in the refrigerator where they can be kept for up to two weeks.

Kitchen Prescription

Put the Squeeze on Disease! Using orange juice as a base for smoothies is a fast and easy way to marry the benefits of these fruits to those of other cancer fighters such as berries, cherries, and peaches and make it into a delicious drink of protection! Also try our Orange, Watercress, and Red Onion Salad.

Papaya

Tropical fruits thought to be native to the Americas, papayas are also a wonderful source of carotenoids.

✤ **Serving.** One raw papaya (approximately 11 ounces) contains 120 calories, 2 grams protein, 30 grams carbohydrates, 0.5 gram fat, no cholesterol, and 2.9 grams dietary fiber. The same serving provides 62 percent of the RDA of vitamin A (615 RE), 317 percent of the RDA of vitamin C (190 mg), 6 percent of the RDA of calcium (75 mg), and 790 milligrams potassium.

✤ **Selecting and storing.** Look for brightly colored papayas that give slightly to palm pressure. Slightly green papayas will ripen quickly at room temperature, especially if placed in a paper bag. Refrigerate completely ripe fruit and use as soon as possible. Ripe papaya is best eaten raw, whereas slightly green fruit can be cooked like a vegetable.

Kitchen Prescription

Papayas are known as a digestive aid because they contain an enzyme called papain.

Peaches

Widely planted across the Eastern seaboard by the early settlers, many botanists thought the fruit to be indigenous to the United States. The peach is the third most popular of all fruits grown here and comes in numerous varieties. Peaches provide two classes of cancer-fighters: flavonoids and carotenoids.

❖ **Serving.** One peach (approximately 4 ounces) contains 37 calories, 0.7 gram protein, 9.7 grams carbohydrates, 0.1 gram fat, no cholesterol, and 1.5 grams dietary fiber. The same serving provides 47 percent of the RDA of vitamin A (465 RE), 19 percent of the RDA of vitamin C (1.7 mg), and 8 percent of the RDA of niacin (1.5 mg).

❖ **Selecting and storing.** Peaches are available from May to October in most regions of the country. Look for fragrant fruit that gives slightly to palm pressure. Avoid those with any signs of greening.

 Kitchen Prescription

Warm (or Cool) and Fuzzy! Try our Frozen Gingered Peach Yogurt Pie for a delicious and light dessert filled with flavonoids.

Peas

Members of the bean family and dating back as far as 9700 B.C., peas were used by Gregor Mendel in groundbreaking genetic experiments that demonstrated how genes are passed from generation to generation. Peas also provide flavonoids to help protect DNA from damage and phytoestrogens that interfere with estrogen's ability to interact with and encourage the growth of certain tumors.

✤ **Serving.** One-half cup of cooked peas contains 67 calories, 4.3 grams protein, 12.5 grams carbohydrates, 0.2 gram fat, no cholesterol, and 3 grams dietary fiber. The same serving provides 25 percent of the RDA of folate (50.7 mcg), 19 percent of the RDA of vitamin C (1.7 mg), and 8 percent of the RDA of niacin (1.5 mg).

✤ **Selecting and storing.** Choose fresh peas that have plump, bright green pods. The peas inside should be glossy, crunchy, and sweet. Refrigerate peas in their pods in a plastic bag for no more than two to three days. Store dried peas in a cool, dry place.

 Kitchen Prescription

Peas to Please! Whether you're partial to the frozen, dented variety or prefer garden-fresh peas, they are a great addition to your meals. Try our Crisp Asian Salad with snow peas.

Peppers

Thought by seventeenth-century Europeans to cure digestive problems and ulcers, peppers have been confirmed by modern medicine to contain numerous compounds that have beneficial effects on the digestive system. Many varieties of peppers exist, including banana peppers, red bell, yellow bell, green bell, chili, cayenne, jalapeño, habanero, and Scotch bonnet.

✤ **Serving.** One-half cup of red bell pepper contains 14 calories, 0.5 gram protein, 3.2 grams carbohydrates, 0.1 gram fat, no

cholesterol, and 1.8 grams dietary fiber. The same serving provides 11 percent of the RDA of folate (22.2 mcg), 44 percent of
the RDA of vitamin C (26.1 mg), 35 percent of the RDA of vitamin B_6 (0.7 mg), 17 percent of the RDA of niacin (3.3 mg), 18
percent of the RDA of thiamin (0.2 mg), 14 percent of the RDA
of magnesium (54.5 mg), 19 percent of the RDA of iron (2.8
mg), and 844 milligrams potassium.

✤ **Selecting and storing.** Choose peppers that are firm, feel
heavy for their size, and have a brightly colored, shiny skin. Avoid
those that are limp or shriveled or that have soft or bruised spots.
Store peppers in a plastic bag in the refrigerator for up to a week.

 Kitchen Prescription

Depending on the color, peppers contain a variety of cancer-fighting
compounds, including p-coumaric acid, chlorogenic acid, beta-
cryptoxanthin (red peppers), and lycopene (red peppers).

Plums

Relatives of the almond and used to make prunes, plums are versatile fruits with several varieties.

✤ **Serving.** One plum contains 36 calories, 0.6 gram protein,
8.6 grams carbohydrates, 0.5 gram fat, no cholesterol, and 1 gram
dietary fiber. The same serving provides 11 percent of the RDA
of vitamin C (6.3 mg), 5 percent of the RDA of vitamin B_6 (0.1
mg), 7 percent of the RDA of thiamin (0.1 mg), 6 percent of the
RDA of riboflavin (0.1 mg), and 113 milligrams potassium.

✤ **Selecting and storing.** Fresh plums are available from May
to late October. Choose firm fruit that gives slightly to palm pressure. Store in a cool, dry place.

Kitchen Prescription

Try our unique Grilled Fruit Kebabs for a hot take on this cool fruit that's rich in flavonoids.

Pomegranates

Unusual fruits with bright red juice and many seeds, the name *pomegranate* comes from two French words, *pomme* and *granate*, literally meaning "apple with many seeds." These unique fruits provide a healthy dose of anthocyanins to help reduce inflammatory cytokines to fight cancer (learn more in Chapter 4).

✣ **Serving.** One pomegranate (approximately 5.5 ounces) contains 104 calories, 1.5 grams protein, 26.5 grams carbohydrates, 0.5 gram fat, no cholesterol, and 1 gram dietary fiber. The same serving provides 16 percent of the RDA of vitamin C (9.4 mg) and 399 milligrams potassium.

✣ **Selecting and storing.** In the United States pomegranates are available in October and November. Choose those that are heavy for their size and have a bright, fresh color and blemish-free skin. You can refrigerate them for up to two months or store them in a cool, dark place for up to a month.

 Kitchen Prescription

With a red stain you won't forget (or ever get out!), pomegranates provide anthocyanins. Sprinkle these juicy buds over your favorite cereal.

Pumpkin

A flowering vegetable and member of the melon and squash (Cucurbitaceae) family, the pumpkin is a powerhouse of carotenoids to be enjoyed year-round.

✤ **Serving.** One-half cup of canned pumpkin contains 41 calories, 1.3 grams protein, 9.9 grams carbohydrates, 0.3 gram fat, no cholesterol, and 3.6 grams dietary fiber. The same serving provides 269 percent of the RDA of vitamin A (2,691 RE), 8 percent of the RDA of folate (15 mcg), 9 percent of the RDA of vitamin C (5.1 mg), 7 percent of the RDA of magnesium (28 mg), 11 percent of the RDA of iron (1.7 mg), and 251 milligrams potassium.

✤ **Selecting and storing.** Fresh pumpkins are available in the fall and winter, and some specimens have weighed in at well over one hundred pounds. In general, however, the flesh from smaller sizes will be more tender and succulent. Choose pumpkins that are free from blemishes and heavy for their size. Store whole pumpkins at room temperature for up to a month or refrigerate for up to three months. Canned pumpkin is a great way to enjoy these gorgeous gourds year-round—add to smoothies, breads, and muffins.

 Kitchen Prescription

Can't think of a way to eat pumpkin except in a pie? Try our Pumpkin Buckwheat Flapjacks, or try incorporating this great gourd into a smoothie with almond milk and cinnamon.

Raspberries

Typically red, raspberries also come in other colors such as purple, yellow, amber, and black.

❖ **Serving.** One cup of raspberries contains 61 calories, 1.2 grams protein, 14.3 grams carbohydrates, 0.7 gram fat, no cholesterol, and 8 grams dietary fiber. The same serving provides 16 percent of the RDA of folate (32 mcg), 51 percent of the RDA of vitamin C (30.8 mg), 6 percent of the RDA of magnesium (22 mg), and 5 percent of the RDA of iron (0.7 mg).

❖ **Selecting and storing.** Raspberries are available from May through November. Choose brightly colored, plump berries without the hull. If the hulls are still attached, the berries were picked too early and will undoubtedly be tart. Avoid soft, shriveled, or moldy berries. Store them in a dry container in the refrigerator for two to three days. If necessary, rinse berries lightly just before serving.

 Kitchen Prescription

Raspberries also contain ellagic acid to disarm carcinogens and protect against cell mutations that can lead to cancer.

Rice

Originating in southeast Asia, rice is the second most highly consumed food in the world. It provides vitamin B_6, along with phenols and other phytonutrients.

❖ **Serving.** One-half cup of medium-grain brown rice contains 110 calories, 2.3 grams protein, 23 grams carbohydrates, 0.8 gram fat, no cholesterol, and 1.7 grams dietary fiber. The same serving provides 10 percent of the RDA of vitamin B_6 (0.2 mg), 5 percent of the RDA of niacin (1.0 mg), 67 percent of the RDA of thiamin (1.0 mg), 11 percent of the RDA of magnesium (43 mg), and 3 percent of the RDA of iron (0.5 mg).

❖ **Selecting and storing.** Brown rice, due to the presence of bran, is subject to rancidity, which limits its shelf life to only about six months.

 Kitchen Prescription

Don't forget to get brown rice that's still intact so it has its cancer-fighting bran and germ layers.

Soybeans

Members of the bean family and a complete protein source, soybeans are a main staple of the Asian diet. Many varieties of soy foods exist. Edamame are soybeans in their shell, which can be purchased in the frozen section of your grocery store in the pod or in the refrigerated case, cooked, and out of their shells. Tempeh is soybean curd that has a meaty texture and can also be found in the refrigerator case. Textured vegetable protein (TVP) is processed soy that has the consistency of ground meat. It can be used in chilis, sauces, soups, or anywhere you would use ground meat. It's available in either the dry section of your grocery or in the freezer section. All soy foods take on the flavors you cook them with, so make liberal use of those phytonutrient herbs and spices when cooking with soy products.

❖ **Serving.** One-quarter block of tofu (approximately 4 ounces) contains 90 calories, 9.4 grams protein, 2.2 grams carbohydrates, 5.4 grams fat, no cholesterol, and 1.4 grams dietary fiber. The same serving provides 30 percent of the RDA of magnesium (120 mg), 41 percent of the RDA of iron (6.2 mg), and 10 percent of the RDA of calcium (122 mg).

❖ **Selecting and storing.** Tofu is very perishable and should be refrigerated for no more than a week. If it's packaged in water, drain it and cover it with fresh water; change the water daily. Tofu can be frozen for up to three months. Read individual soy foods for specific storing instructions.

 Kitchen Prescription

Soybeans contain an array of phytonutrients, including isoflavones, such as diadzein and genistein, that interfere with estrogen's ability to fuel tumor growth.

Spinach

A leafy green native of Asia, spinach was taken to Europe by the Moors when they conquered Spain in the eighth century. You'll find carotenoids, lutein, zeaxanthin, and chlorophyll in this vegetable.

❖ **Serving.** One-half cup of cooked spinach contains 21 calories, 2.7 grams protein, 3.4 grams carbohydrates, 0.2 gram fat, no cholesterol, and 2.1 grams dietary fiber. The same serving provides 74 percent of the RDA of vitamin A (737 RE), 66 percent of the RDA of folate (131.2 mcg), 20 percent of the RDA of magnesium (78.3 mg), 21 percent of the RDA of iron (3.2 mg), and 10 percent of the RDA of calcium (122.4 mg).

❖ **Selecting and storing.** Fresh spinach is available year-round. Choose leaves that are crisp and dark green with a nice fresh fragrance. Avoid those that are limp or damaged or that have yellow spots. You can refrigerate spinach in a plastic bag for up to three days. Spinach, which is usually very gritty, must be thoroughly rinsed.

 Kitchen Prescription

Because most of the compounds in spinach are fat soluble, heating it up and adding some oil unlocks its power. Try our Eggplant, Spinach, and Garbanzo Bean Curry.

Squash

A flowering vegetable native to the Americas, squash varieties include acorn, spaghetti, zucchini, crookneck, and butternut.

❖ **Serving.** One-half cup of baked acorn squash contains 57 calories, 1.1 grams protein, 14.9 grams carbohydrates, 0.1 gram fat, no cholesterol, and 2.9 grams dietary fiber. The same serving provides 18 percent of the RDA of vitamin C (11 mg), 13 percent of the RDA of thiamin (0.2 mg), 11 percent of the RDA of magnesium (44 mg), and 445.7 milligrams potassium.

❖ **Selecting and storing.** Although most varieties are available year-round, winter squash is best from early fall through winter. Choose squash that are heavy for their size and have a hard, deep-colored rind that's free of blemishes or moldy or soft spots. Winter squash can be kept in a cool, dark place for a month or more, depending on the variety.

Kitchen Prescription

All types of squash are potent parcels of carotenoids, including alpha-carotene and beta-carotene.

Strawberries

This is the most popular American berry, with more than seventy nutrient-rich varieties. Strawberries contain a long list of anti-cancer nutrients, including ellagic acid, lycopene, p-coumaric acid, chlorogenic acid, kaempferol, and anthocyanins.

❖ **Serving.** One cup of raw strawberries contains 45 calories, 1 gram protein, 10.5 grams carbohydrates, 0.6 gram fat, no cholesterol, and 2.9 grams dietary fiber. The same serving provides 13 percent of the RDA of folate (26.4 mcg), 141 percent of the RDA of vitamin C (84.5 mg), 4 percent of the RDA of iron (0.6 mg), and 247 milligrams potassium.

❖ **Selecting and storing.** Fresh strawberries are available year-round in many regions of the country, with the peak season running from April to June. Choose brightly colored, plump berries that still have their leaves attached. Avoid soft, shriveled, or moldy berries. Do not wash strawberries until you're ready to use them; you can store them in a dry container in the refrigerator for two to three days.

Kitchen Prescription

Try strawberries in our Hydrating Smoothie or in our Banana Berry Cooler.

Tea

Used by the ancient Chinese, the Greeks, medieval herbalists, and scholars of the Enlightenment for medicinal purposes, black tea, green tea, and oolong tea come from the *Camellia sinensis* plant. Tea contains potent cancer-fighting compounds, including tannins, catechins, and polyphenols. (Refer back to Chapter 4 to learn about the role of epigallocatechin gallate.)

❉ **Serving.** A six-ounce cup of black tea contains 2 calories, no protein, 0.5 gram carbohydrates, no fat, no cholesterol, and no dietary fiber. The same serving provides 5 percent of the RDA of folate (1 mcg).

❉ **Selecting and storing.** Store tea bags or loose tea in an airtight container in a cool, dry place.

 Kitchen Prescription

Drink to Your Health! Steep your tea for two minutes to maximize health benefits.

Tomatoes

Thought to have originated in South America, tomatoes were taken to Europe by Spanish explorers in the 1500s. One of the most famous cancer-fighting phytonutrients, lycopene, is found abundantly in tomatoes.

❉ **Serving.** One ripe tomato (approximately 4.3 ounces) contains 24 calories, 1.1 grams protein, 5.3 grams carbohydrates, 0.3 gram fat, no cholesterol, and 1.3 grams dietary fiber. The same serving provides 14 percent of the RDA of vitamin A (139 RE), 6 percent of the RDA of folate (11.6 mcg), 36 percent of the

RDA of vitamin C (21.6 mg), and 5 percent of the RDA of iron (0.8 mg).

✤ **Selecting and storing.** Choose firm, well-shaped fruit that are fragrant and richly colored (for their variety). They should be free from blemishes, feel heavy for their size, and give slightly to pressure. Ripe tomatoes should be stored at room temperature and used within a few days, because cold temperatures make the flesh pulpy and diminishes their flavor.

 Kitchen Prescription

Lycopene, as a fat-soluble compound, loves to get heated up. So start the tomato sauce!

Watercress

A member of the crucifer (mustard) family of vegetables, this naturally aquatic plant flourishes when grown hydroponically (in nutrient solutions). It is cultivated worldwide and can be found growing naturally in streams or other moving water.

✤ **Serving.** One-half cup of chopped, raw watercress contains 2 calories, 0.4 gram protein, 0.2 gram carbohydrates, a trace of fat, no cholesterol, and 0.4 gram dietary fiber. The same serving provides 8 percent of the RDA of vitamin A (80 RE) and 12 percent of the RDA of vitamin C (7.3 mg).

✤ **Selecting and storing.** Watercress is available year-round and is customarily sold in small bouquets. Choose crisp leaves with deep, vibrant color. There should be no sign of yellowing or wilting. Refrigerate the bouquet in a plastic bag (or stem-down in a glass of water covered with a plastic bag) for up to five days. Wash the greens and shake them dry just before using.

Kitchen Prescription

Try this indole-rich veggie in our Orange, Watercress, and Red Onion Salad.

Watermelon

A native of Africa, the watermelon spread to Asia and the Mediterranean because of its usefulness as a source of potable liquid. It provides vitamin B_6 for cellular defense and is the red member of the carotenoid family, providing lycopene.

❖ **Serving.** One cup of watermelon contains 51 calories, 1 gram protein, 11.5 grams carbohydrates, 0.7 gram fat, no cholesterol, and 0.6 gram dietary fiber. The same serving provides 6 percent of the RDA of vitamin A (59 RE), 26 percent of the RDA of vitamin C (15.4 mg), 10 percent of the RDA of vitamin B_6 (0.2 mg), 7 percent of the RDA of thiamin (0.1 mg), 5 percent of the RDA of magnesium (18 mg), and 185 milligrams potassium.

❖ **Selecting and storing.** Watermelons are available from May to September, though they're at their peak from mid-June to late August. Look for symmetrical melons without any flat sides. Depending on the variety, the shape can be round or oval. A hollow thump when slapped indicates ripeness. Cut watermelon should always be tightly wrapped, refrigerated, and used within a day or so.

Kitchen Prescription

Try this medicinal melon in our Hydrating Smoothie.

Wheat

One of the oldest grains cultivated, wheat is available in numerous forms, including berries, cracked wheat, bulgur grits, shredded wheat, unprocessed bran (or miller's bran), wheat germ, rolled wheat flakes, puffed wheat, Cream of Wheat, and wheat flour. As a grain, it provides ferulic acid.

❖ **Serving.** One slice of whole-wheat bread contains 90 calories, 4 grams protein, 15 grams carbohydrates, 1 gram fat, no cholesterol, and 3 grams dietary fiber. The same serving also provides 2 percent of the RDA for folate (4.1 mcg), 6 percent of the RDA for niacin (1.2 mg), 6 percent of the RDA for thiamin (0.09 mg), and 2 percent of the RDA for riboflavin (0.04 mg).

❖ **Selecting and storing.** Whole-wheat flour contains part of the grain's germ and turns rancid quickly because of the oil in the germ. Refrigerate or freeze the flour, tightly wrapped, and use it as soon as possible.

 Kitchen Prescription

Go with the (Whole) Grain! Don't forget to look for the words *whole grain* on wheat products to ensure you're getting the important germ and bran layers that stock the cancer-fighting arsenal.

Yogurt

Yogurt has been a culinary staple in Asia, the Middle East, and Eastern Europe for centuries. In 1931, commercial production of the cultured dairy product began in the United States. Yogurt contains probiotics when the label reads "contains live and active cultures."

❖ **Serving.** One cup of plain, low-fat yogurt contains 144 calories, 11.9 grams protein, 16 grams carbohydrates, 3.5 grams fat, 14 milligrams cholesterol, and no fiber. The same serving provides 64 percent of the RDA of vitamin B_{12} (1.28 mcg), 35 percent of the RDA of calcium (415 mg), 10 percent of the RDA of magnesium (40 mg), and 531 milligrams potassium.

❖ **Selecting and storing.** Always buy yogurt with live and active cultures for the maximum nutritional benefit.

 Kitchen Prescription

Get your yogurt in our Frozen Gingered Peach Yogurt Pie.

So far, we've examined the various nutritional elements in different foods and diets. Next, you'll learn what herbs and spices you should be stocking in your kitchen.

Healing Herbs and Spices

THE SMELL OF GINGER wafting through Chinatown or the scent of oregano at your local pizzeria may be an ingredient in the recipe to reducing cancer risk. Not only do these herbs and spices add flavor, but they are packed with—of course—phytonutrients! The liberal use of fragrant spices and herbs is not a new concept. For centuries these flavor enhancers have been used to boost enjoyment of cuisine, treat illnesses, and prevent spoilage.

Savoring Flavor

In ancient times, people prized spices more highly than gold or jewels. In today's world of high-sodium and high-fat processed foods, consumers are turning to herbs and spices to add flavor and zest to their meals. Using nature's flavor enhancers delivers an abundance of cancer fighters while eliminating added calories and salt. Researchers at the Cytokine Research Laboratory, Department of Experimental Therapeutics at the University of Texas, uniquely describe this as the "reasoning for seasoning." Remember that in Chapter 4 you learned how each of the phytonutrients works as part of a team to fight cancer? Take a look at Table 6.1, which illustrates some of the cancer-fighting herbs and spices and

TABLE 6.1 Cancer-Fighting Herbs and Spices

Herb/Spice Family	Herb/Spice Members	Phytonutrients
Labiatae (mint) family	Basil, mint, oregano, sage, rosemary, thyme	Terpenoids, menthol, chlorophyll
Umbelliferae (carrot) family	Anise, caraway, carrots, celeriac, celery, chervil, cilantro, coriander, cumin, dill, fennel, parsley, parsnips	Carotenoids, beta-carotene, alpha-carotene, beta-cryptoxanthin, zeaxanthin, lutein, chlorophyll
Zingiberaceae (ginger) family	Ginger, turmeric	Curcumin, gingerols, zingibain

the phytonutrients responsible for their delicious protective abilities.

A Spice Rack of Protection

Unlike herbs, which come from the leaves of plants, spices are made from the bud, bark, fruit, seed, or root. Although research of the healing powers of spices is relatively new, what scientists have discovered thus far has been impressive. Rich in phytonutrients and antioxidants, spices have been found to reduce cholesterol, keep the arteries clear, stabilize blood sugar, and fight cancer. As with the other plants we eat, the colors tell us how these flavor-enhancers work in our bodies to prevent cancer.

🍎 **Kitchen Prescription**

Boost the flavor of spices by toasting them briefly in a dry skillet until slightly brown and aromatic.

Most spices, including cinnamon, bay leaves, allspice, and cloves, help to protect us from cancer through their antioxidant action and beneficial effects on blood sugar. As we discussed in Chapter 3 with the glycemic index, keeping blood sugar stable may be an important factor in preventing cancer and its growth. Let's take a look at the individual spices to include in your rack and some of the recipes from Chapter 9 in which they're incorporated.

Allspice. This is the dried, unripe berry of *Pimenta dioica*, an evergreen tree in the myrtle family. After drying, the berries are small, dark brown balls just a little larger than peppercorns. Allspice comes from Jamaica, Mexico, and Honduras. Pungent and fragrant, it is not a blend of "all spices," but its taste and aroma remind many people of a mix of cloves, cinnamon, and nutmeg. Allspice is used in Jamaican jerk seasoning and in Jamaican soups, stews, and curries. It also appears in pickling spice, spiced tea mixes, cakes, cookies, and pies.

Anise. A gray-brown, oval seed from *Pimpinella anisum*, a plant in the carrot (Umbelliferae) family, anise is related to caraway, dill, cumin, and fennel. Spain and Mexico are the sources for anise, although it is native to the Middle East. Europeans and Americans use anise in cakes, cookies, and sweet breads; in the Middle East and India, it is used in soups and stews.

Bay Leaves. Bay leaves come from the sweet bay or laurel tree, known botanically as *Laurus nobilis*. The elliptical leaves of the trees are green, glossy, and grow up to three inches long. Grown in the Mediterranean region and a staple in American kitchens, bay leaves are used in soups, stews, and meat and vegetable dishes. The leaves also flavor classic French dishes such as bouillabaisse.

 Kitchen Prescription

Taste bay leaves in our Mustard Baked Salmon with Lentils.

Cinnamon. Cinnamon is the dried bark of various trees (*Cinnamomum*) from the laurel family. The cinnamon used in North America is from the cassia tree, which is grown in Vietnam, China, Indonesia, and Central America. Cinnamon has a sweet, woody fragrance in both ground and stick forms and enhances the taste of vegetables and fruits.

 Kitchen Prescription

Our Grilled Fruit Kebabs are a delicious example of how to use cinnamon.

Cloves. Cloves are the rich, brown, dried, unopened flower buds of *Syzygium aromaticum*, an evergreen tree in the myrtle family. The name comes from the French *clou* meaning "nail." Cloves come from Madagascar, Brazil, Penang, and Ceylon and are strong, pungent, and sweet.

Cumin. This is the pale green seed of *Cuminum cyminum*, a small herb in the carrot family. The seed is uniformly elliptical and deeply furrowed. It is frequently used in Mexican dishes and has a distinctive, slightly bitter, yet warm flavor.

Fennel. This seed is the oval, green or yellowish-brown dried fruit of *Foeniculum vulgare*, a member of the carrot family. Fennel goes well with fish and is used in some curry powder mixes. It has an aniselike flavor but is more aromatic, sweeter, and less pungent.

Ginger. A member of the Zingiberaceae family—which includes turmeric—ginger comes mainly from Jamaica, India, Africa, and China. With a peppery, slightly sweet flavor and a spicy, pungent aroma, this extremely versatile root has long been a mainstay in Asian and Indian cooking. It found its way early on into European foods as well. Young ginger, often called spring ginger, has a pale, thin skin that requires no peeling. Mature ginger has a tough skin that must be peeled away to use the delicate flesh just under the surface.

 Kitchen Prescription

Try upping your ginger intake with our Tummy-Soothing Smoothie.

Saffron. The stigma of *Crocus sativus*, a flowering plant in the crocus family and native to the Mediterranean, saffron is the world's most expensive spice. More than 225,000 stigmas must be hand-picked to produce one pound of spice. In its pure form, saffron is a mass of compressed, threadlike, dark orange strands. Primarily cultivated in Spain, saffron is used in French bouillabaisse, Spanish paella, and many Middle Eastern dishes. It has a spicy, pungent, and bitter flavor with a sharp and penetrating odor.

 Kitchen Prescription

Try this pricey spice in our Steamed Mussels with Saffron Sauce.

Turmeric. Turmeric comes from the root of *Curcuma longa*, a leafy plant in the ginger family. The root, or rhizome, has a tough brown skin and bright orange flesh. Ground turmeric comes from fingers that extend from the root. It is boiled or steamed and then dried and ground. India is the world's primary producer of turmeric, but it is also grown in China and Indonesia. Turmeric is a necessary ingredient of curry powder and is used extensively in Indian dishes—including lentil and meat dishes—and in southeast Asian cooking. Turmeric is mildly aromatic and has scents of orange or ginger. It has a pungent, bitter flavor.

 Kitchen Prescription

Get turmeric in our Eggplant, Spinach, and Garbanzo Bean Curry.

Herbs for Health

Prior to the discovery of modern pharmaceuticals, both Europeans and Americans relied on herbs to treat illness and promote health. Researchers now know that the phytonutrients in herbs provide a range of health benefits, including working as part of your cancer-fighting food team. Although numerous healing herbs exist, we will focus on some of the most common culinary varieties that bring aroma to your kitchen and an added dose of health to your meals.

Basil. A bright green, leafy plant (*Ocimum basilicum*) in the mint (Labiatae) family, basil is grown primarily in the United States, France, and the Mediterranean. Basil is widely used in Italian cuisine and is often paired with tomatoes. It is also used in Thai cooking. Basil has a sweet, herbal bouquet and its name means "be fragrant."

Kitchen Prescription

Try our Mediterranean Gateau starring this herb.

Cilantro. The leaf of the young coriander plant (*Coriandrum sativum*), cilantro is an herb in the carrot family that is similar to anise. Grown in California and traditionally used in Middle Eastern, Mexican, and Asian cooking, cilantro's taste is a fragrant mix of parsley and citrus.

 Kitchen Prescription

Try this unique-flavored herb in our Rice, Corn, and Bean Medley with Cilantro, Coriander, and Cumin.

Dill. This tall, feathery annual (*Anethum graveolens*), is in the carrot family. Both dill seed and weed (dried leaves) come from the same plant and are widely used in pickling as well as in German, Russian, and Scandinavian dishes. The dill seed flavor is clean, pungent, and reminiscent of caraway; dill weed has a similar but mellower and fresher flavor.

Marjoram. Marjoram is the gray-green leaf of *Majorana hortensis*, a low-growing member of the mint family. Often mistaken for oregano, marjoram has a delicate, sweet, pleasant flavor with a slightly bitter undertone.

Mint. Mint is the dried leaf of a perennial herb in the Labiatae family. There are two important species, *Mentha spicata L.* (spearmint) and *Mentha piperita L.* (peppermint).

Kitchen Prescription

Try our Chopped Mediterranean Salad, which includes several members of the mint family.

Mediterranean Oregano. This is the dried leaf of *Origanum vulgare L.*, a perennial herb in the mint family. Mexican oregano is the dried leaf of one of several plants of the *Lippia* genus. Grown in California and New Mexico, as well as the Mediterranean region, oregano is the spice that gives pizza its characteristic flavor. It is also usually used in chili powder. It has a pungent odor and flavor, with the Mexican variety being a bit stronger than Mediterranean oregano.

Parsley. Parsley (*Petroselinum crispum*) is another member of the carrot family and is commonly used as a flavoring and garnish. Although more than thirty varieties of this herb exist, the most popular are curly-leaf parsley and the more strongly flavored Italian or flat-leaf parsley.

Kitchen Prescription

Our Tabbouleh Primavera makes liberal use of parsley.

Rosemary. This is an herb in the mint family. A small evergreen shrub native to the Mediterranean, the leaves of *Rosmarinus officinalis* resemble curved pine needles. Today it is widely produced in France, Spain, and Portugal and has a distinctive tealike aroma and a piney flavor. Rosemary contains rosmarinic acid, among other phytonutrients that help to reduce inflammatory factors involved with the development of heart disease and other chronic illnesses.

Sage. An herb from an evergreen shrub (*Salvia officinalis*) in the mint family, sage's long, grayish-green leaves take on a velvety, cottonlike texture when rubbed (meaning they are ground lightly and passed through a coarse sieve). Grown primarily in the United States as well as Dalmatia and Albania, sage has a fragrant aroma and an astringent but warm flavor. The name *sage* comes from the Latin word *salvia* meaning "to save."

Thyme. Thyme is the leaf of a low-growing shrub in the mint family called *Thymus vulgaris*. Its tiny grayish-green leaves rarely grow longer than one-fourth of an inch. For use as a condiment, thyme leaves are dried, then chopped or ground. Grown in southern Europe, including France, Spain, and Portugal, thyme is also indigenous to the Mediterranean. It has a subtle, dry aroma and a slightly minty flavor.

Perfect Pairings

Now that we have explored some of the healing properties of herbs and spices, let's take a look at the flavor combinations that please the palette. Don't be afraid to experiment and create your own blends to design savory and healthy meals.

* **Poultry.** Rosemary and thyme; tarragon, marjoram, and garlic; cumin, bay leaf, and saffron (or turmeric); ginger, cinnamon, and allspice; curry powder and thyme
* **Fish and seafood.** Cumin and oregano; tarragon, thyme, parsley, and garlic; thyme, fennel, saffron, and red pepper; ginger, sesame, and white pepper; cilantro, parsley, cumin, and garlic
* **Beans.** Marjoram and rosemary; caraway and dry mustard
* **Broccoli.** Ginger and garlic; sesame and nutmeg
* **Cabbage.** Celery seeds and dill; curry powder and nutmeg

* **Carrots.** Cinnamon and nutmeg; ginger
* **Corn.** Chili powder and cumin; dill
* **Peas.** Anise; rosemary and marjoram
* **Spinach.** Curry powder and ginger; nutmeg and garlic
* **Summer squash.** Mint and parsley; tarragon and garlic
* **Winter squash.** Cinnamon and nutmeg; allspice and red pepper
* **Tomatoes.** Basil and rosemary; cinnamon and ginger
* **Potatoes.** Dill and parsley; caraway; nutmeg and chives
* **Rice.** Chili powder and cumin; curry powder, ginger, and coriander; cinnamon, cardamom, and cloves
* **Pasta.** Basil, rosemary, and parsley; cumin, turmeric, and red pepper; oregano and thyme

Now that you've seen how the various foods, herbs, and spices work together, the next chapter gives you some strategies and tips for stocking your kitchen with the healthiest ingredients to improve your quality of life and chances for prevention or recovery.

7

Stocking Your Pantry

WITH A PLETHORA of culinary choices to make, selecting the right ingredients to stock your pantry to help prevent or cope with cancer can be a daunting task. In this chapter, you will learn how to decipher food labels and shop for the healthiest ingredients, what claims on food products mean, and how to spot those sneaky health-harming ingredients found in so many packaged foods.

Tips for Smart Shopping

Understanding the science behind how foods can protect us is only useful if we can translate that information into our grocery carts and ultimately onto our tables. Because most of us spend a substantial amount of time at the grocery store (84 percent of consumers prepare home-cooked meals at least three times a week), it is critical to navigate the supermarket smorgasbord to sleuth out the healthiest products. Take a look at the following simple tips to help you stay on track when shopping, while still enjoying some delicious foods.

Before You Go to the Store

Smart shopping begins before you leave the house. Being unprepared leads to multiple trips, unwanted purchases, and often unhealthy choices finding their way into your shopping cart. Stray from your list only if the item is a healthy one. If a junior shopper vying for the candy aisle accompanies you, have him or her explore the produce section and choose a unique fruit or vegetable (such as a persimmon, a pomegranate, or a kiwi) to try to foster good health habits.

In addition, make sure to eat first, then shop. Shopping when you're hungry is a surefire way to end up straying from your list and succumbing to unhealthy choices. Having a small snack will help you to avoid temptations that will wind up in your cupboard and on your waist.

How to Shop

Instead of buying on impulse, rely on your list. Studies have shown gender differences when it comes to shopping: women tend to browse, whereas men tend to know what they're looking for and get it. So, ladies, don't be afraid to shop like a man.

Another useful tip is to become a perimeter shopper. The exterior of the store contains many of the whole foods we have described for optimum health. Spend most of your time shopping for fresh produce, seafood, lean meats, and dairy. When choosing dairy, opt for lower-calorie products like nonfat yogurt, part-skim mozzarella cheese, or low-fat fresh and soft cheeses as opposed to aged, hard cheeses like cheddar, which rack up 100 calories for each one-ounce cube.

Finally, be sure to read labels. There is a great deal of variation in the health value of different brands of foods, so it's important to pause and compare choices. Look at ingredient lists, calories and sugar, type of grain used (whole grains versus refined), and type of oils used (olive oil or canola oil versus partially hydrogenated vegetable oil). We will demystify the food label later in this chapter.

What to Buy

Remember all those healing herbs and spices you read about in Chapter 6? The condiment aisle is full of flavor and is a great way to add zest to your healthy foods. Purchase high-quality cooking oils like extra-virgin olive oil, sesame oil, expeller-pressed canola oil, and other liquid vegetable oils for sautés, dressings, and marinades. Buy mustard, vinegars, horseradish, dried herbs, and spices that add virtually no calories and lots of flavor to all varieties of foods. Also, don't be afraid to just go nuts! Instead of chips, pretzels, and other nutrient-void snack foods, opt for roasted nuts and seeds—which are full of minerals, good-quality fats, and other health-promoting nutrients. Just be sure to watch your portion size: a quarter cup of almonds, for example, contains 170 calories.

Frozen vegetables, fruits, seafood, and poultry are a more economical way to eat healthy. Having a freezer stocked with these staples ensures you can whip up a delicious meal in minutes. In short, put the freeze on disease! Try frozen fruits like blueberries, mixed berries, and cherries for smoothies and fruit-based desserts. Opt for frozen edamame (soybeans in their pods) for an easy appetizer or Asian meal. Bagged, mixed veggies are perfect for making vegetable soups like minestrone; research shows that the nutrient content is equal to or greater than that of fresh vegetables—which can lose many vitamins in shipping and handling. By adding a few additional ingredients, frozen foods can provide you with a healthy base for many of your meals.

Another easy tip to follow when shopping is to color your cart. When you look in your shopping cart, the vast majority of your food selection should be fruits and vegetables to reach the goal of at least five to nine servings a day. Look for those colors we listed in Chapter 5 and build your meals around them. Blueberry smoothies, hearty red marinara sauces, green salads, and multicolor vegetable soups should be your mainstays.

What to Limit

Beware of not-so-healthy "health" foods. Sports drinks and energy bars are not much more than sugar fortified with vitamins and minerals, each packing a whopping 200-plus calories per serving. The same goes for desserts and snack foods that are labeled "organic." These are no better than their "conventional" counterparts when it comes to nutrition. Also, avoid the deli. Although many deli foods are marketed as fresh, most are processed red meats or poultry, which contain carcinogenic preservatives called sodium nitrites.

Finally, don't drown in the beverage aisle. Good old H_2O and flavored waters without calories are a smart choice. Avoid sugary, high-calorie iced teas; pseudosmoothies; sweetened milks; and coffee beverages. They add up quickly but don't necessarily make you feel full.

Understanding Label Lingo

Just about every packaged food made in the United States has a food label indicating serving size, nutritional information, and ingredients. Unfortunately, this critical piece of information is often overlooked, leading to unhealthy food choices that could have easily been avoided. In this section we will explore the important elements of the food label that can become a guide to your health.

Ingredients

Begin with the ingredient list. This is the most detailed information you'll find on what a product contains. You should be looking for answers to these questions:

✤ **Are the fats used in this product healthful or harmful?** Remember to look for foods made with olive, canola, and other healthful oils and to avoid partially hydrogenated oils. This is of particular concern for packaged cereals and other cereal products, cookies, crackers, microwave popcorn, pastries, cake mixes, and chips, but it also applies to salad dressings, soups, frozen foods, and other premade convenience foods.

✤ **Is the product made with whole grains?** If the label does not say "whole," the product is made with refined flour. For example, instead of "wheat flour," look for "whole-wheat flour." This applies for all grain products, including pastas, crackers, and baking mixes.

✤ **How much of each ingredient does the product contain?** The ingredient list is in descending order. The farther down the list you go, the less of the ingredient the product contains.

✤ **Is the product full of sugar?** Avoid products with high fructose corn syrup and fruit sweeteners appearing high on the ingredient list. Although sugars from fresh fruits may be more healthful when consumed in their natural state (for example, as part of a Red Delicious apple), juice concentrate sweeteners have the same effect on blood sugar and the same number of calories as pure sugar.

✤ **How much of the product is actually a fruit or vegetable?** Although the product may be called "Strawberry Crunchies," after reading the food label you may find only a trace of strawberry flavor toward the end of the list. Choose foods that are nutrient-dense, and stay away from those that are merely empty calories.

Serving Size

Serving sizes are based on the amount of food people typically eat. However, many products contain multiple servings per package. Individual snack foods, for example, may contain 100 calories "per serving," but when you read the number of servings, you find that the energy bar you just ate contains three servings at 100 calories each, totaling 300 calories as opposed to the 100 you thought you were consuming. Serving size doesn't just affect calories; it also affects the amounts of all other nutritional components like fat, sugar, and salt.

Calories and Total Fat

Look at calories and focus on where those calories come from. Use your calories as you would a daily stipend and try to make the most of each. Are your calories coming from good-quality fats and whole grains, or are they derived from sugars, saturated fats, and trans fats? The total fat section of the nutrition panel provides the total amount of fat per serving and also breaks down the types of fat and amount of each. Although trans fats may not be listed yet on many products, you can roughly estimate how much trans fat is in a product with a simple math equation:

Total fat − (saturated fat + monounsaturated fat + polyunsaturated fat) = trans fat

By adding the saturated fat, monounsaturated fat, and polyunsaturated fat together and subtracting them from the total fat, you will determine the grams of trans fat in a specific product. For example, look at Smart Balance popcorn. The total fat is 9 grams. The saturated fat is 3.5 grams, the monounsaturated fat is 2.5 grams, and the polyunsaturated fat is 3 grams.

9 − (3.5 grams saturated fat + 2.5 grams monounsaturated fat + 3 grams polyunsaturated fat) = 0 grams trans fat

However, some products do not reveal the different types of fat they contain. The Food Labeling Act mandates that saturated fat and total fat be disclosed. Monounsaturated fat and polyunsaturated fat do not need listing by the manufacturer. The best way to determine if there is trans fat in a product is to read the ingredient list. Any food that lists "hydrogenated" or "partially hydrogenated vegetable oil" contains trans fat and should be avoided. Talk with your registered dietitian regarding the percentage of calories in your diet that should come from fat, depending on your particular nutrition needs. Beginning in 2006, the federal government will be mandating labeling of trans fats.

Cholesterol

Dietary cholesterol can raise your blood cholesterol level, although not as much as trans fat and saturated fat. Because dietary cholesterol is found only in foods that come from animals, by choosing plenty of fruits, vegetables, and whole grains, you can stay under the daily 300 milligrams recommended by the American Heart Association.

Examining Label Claims

Another aspect of food labeling is label claims. As evidence regarding the relationship between diet and disease becomes more and more apparent, the FDA is allowing claims to be placed on foods to help the consumer make healthier choices. There are three types of claims that can be used for foods and dietary supplements: health claims, nutrient content claims, and structure/function claims. This section gives an overview, but you can visit the FDA website (fda.gov) for more information.

Health Claims

Health claims describe a relationship between a food, food component, or dietary supplement ingredient and its effect on reducing the risk of a particular disease or health-related condition. There are three ways by which the FDA exercises its oversight in determining which health claims may be used in labeling for a food or dietary supplement:

1. The 1990 Nutrition Labeling and Education Act requires the FDA to issue regulations authorizing health claims for foods and dietary supplements after a careful review of the scientific evidence submitted in health claim petitions.
2. The 1997 Food and Drug Administration Modernization Act stipulates that health claims must be based on an authoritative statement of a scientific body of the U.S. government or the National Academy of Sciences. Such claims may be used after submission of a health claim notification to the FDA.
3. The 2003 FDA Consumer Health Information for Better Nutrition Initiative provides for qualified health claims when the quality and strength of the scientific evidence falls below what is required for the FDA to issue an authorizing regulation.

FDA-Approved Health Claims Relating to Cancer. You can find the following list of currently approved health claims from the FDA when shopping for products that may help reduce your risk.

1. **Dietary fat and cancer.** "Development of cancer depends on many factors. A diet low in total fat may reduce the risk of some cancers."
2. **Fiber-containing grain products, fruits, and vegetables and cancer.** "Low-fat diets rich in fiber-containing grain products, fruits, and vegetables may reduce the risk of some types of cancer, a disease associated with many factors."
3. **Fruits and vegetables and cancer.** "Low-fat diets rich in fruits and vegetables (foods that are low in fat and may con-

tain dietary fiber, vitamin A, or vitamin C) may reduce the risk of some types of cancer, a disease associated with many factors. Broccoli is high in vitamins A and C, and it is a good source of dietary fiber."

4. **Whole-grain foods and risk of heart disease and certain cancers.** "Diets rich in whole-grain foods and other plant foods and low in total fat, saturated fat, and cholesterol may reduce the risk of heart disease and some cancers."

Structure/Function Claims

These claims describe the role of a nutrient or dietary ingredient in the normal structure or function of the human body. Examples of structure/function claims include "calcium builds strong bones," "fiber maintains bowel regularity," and "antioxidants maintain cell integrity." You will find these types of claims on "functional foods" that may be fortified, fiber laxatives, and some supplements.

Structure/function claims may also describe a benefit related to a nutrient-deficiency disease (like vitamin C and scurvy), as long as the statement also tells how widespread such a disease is in the United States. The manufacturer is responsible for ensuring the accuracy and truthfulness of these claims; although they are not preapproved by the FDA, they must be truthful and not misleading. If a dietary supplement label includes such a claim, it must state in a "disclaimer" that the FDA has not evaluated the claim. The disclaimer must also state that the product is not intended to "diagnose, treat, cure, or prevent any disease," because only a drug can legally make such a claim.

Now it's time to put all of this information to use in the delicious and healthy meal plans and recipes courtesy of the Healing Gourmet. Bon appétit!

8

My Daily Dose: Meal Plans to Get You Started

You don't have to be a master chef to be a Healing Gourmet. Just let the principles and recipes in this book guide you. We have included recipes that are suited for the culinary novice, those pressed for time, and those who want to gain weight or lose weight—and we do it without sacrificing any flavor. Mealtime should be one of the most enjoyable parts of your day, so let us help you make it healthy.

In this chapter you will find seven-day meal plans for three different calorie levels: 1,500, 2,000, and 2,500. We recognize that readers will have different goals for their overall nutrition. The right calorie level for an individual depends on his or her height, age, activity level, and nutritional goals. For example, if you have recently undergone treatment for cancer and are below a healthy weight, you may need to gain some weight. A 2,000- or 2,500-calorie level may help you achieve this.

On the other hand, you may be overweight and after your treatment you may want to lose a few pounds in a healthy way. For you, 1,500 calories a day may be more appropriate. Your registered dietitian can help you select an appropriate calorie level. However, no matter what that level is, each of these meal plans includes the healthy principles of proper diet. All three menus use the following combination of sources:

* ❖ Lean protein sources (ranging from 17 to 23 percent of total calories)
* ❖ Healthy fats—mostly monounsaturated and polyunsaturated fat (ranging from 30 to 35 percent of total calories)
* ❖ Healthy carbohydrates (ranging from 47 to 52 percent of total calories)

In addition, they all include foods that do the following:

* ❖ Limit the use of saturated fat (to less than 8 percent of total calories)
* ❖ Avoid hydrogenated and partially hydrogenated fats (trans fats)
* ❖ Are low in cholesterol (less than 200 mg/day)
* ❖ Are moderate in sodium (less than 3,000 mg/day)
* ❖ Are high in fiber (a minimum of 25 g/day)

Finally, all of these meals encourage the following healthy practices:

* ❖ Consuming a variety of foods
* ❖ Eating plenty of fruits and vegetables
* ❖ Using whole grains as the main choice for breads, cereals, crackers, and pasta
* ❖ Using whole foods, free-range poultry, and fresh herbs and spices

And, most important, they taste great!

In the menus in this chapter, you'll find meals for breakfast, lunch, and dinner, as well as snacks to eat throughout the day. We also include information about the nutritional content for the day and feature recipes from Chapter 9 (indicated with an asterisk). We have included a "Veg Out" option for dinners, which features a vegetarian alternative to a meat-based meal. While the nutritional content (protein, fat, carbohydrates, and so on) is going to be different in the Veg Out option, non-meat-eaters will find close to the same calorie content. However, always talk with your doctor or health professional to make sure the meal plan and options are right for you.

My Meal Plans: 1,500 Calories

If you are overweight and cancer-free, achieving a healthy weight has the benefit of helping to prevent cancer. In addition, certain cancers, including breast cancer, cause people to gain weight, and this plan is ideal in that situation as well. Always talk with your registered dietitian to decide what is right for you.

Day 1

BREAKFAST
1½ cups old-fashioned oatmeal (cooked)
½ cup raspberries
Spring water

MIDMORNING SNACK
1 cup decaffeinated green tea
½ cup hummus
6 carrot sticks

LUNCH
1 cup lentil soup
1 whole-wheat roll

½ cup cantaloupe
1 cup skim milk

AFTERNOON SNACK
1 ounce natural trail mix

DINNER
1 serving Snapper with Thyme, Tomatoes, and Kalamata
    Olives*
½ cup asparagus
1 cup mixed greens topped with
1½ tablespoons olive oil and vinegar dressing

Veg Out! *Substitute Angel-Hair Arrabiata for the fish dish if you like.*

NIGHTTIME SNACK
1 tablespoon natural peanut butter
4 whole-wheat crackers

Nutrition information: 1,469 calories, 86.9 grams protein or 23
percent, 173.3 grams carbohydrates or 45 percent, 55.9 grams total fat
or 33 percent, 68 milligrams cholesterol, 9.1 grams saturated fat or 6
percent, 1,596 milligrams sodium, 35.6 grams dietary fiber

Day 2

BREAKFAST
Power Shake (1 cup frozen strawberries, ½ banana, ½ cup low-
    fat plain yogurt, and 1 cup skim milk)

MIDMORNING SNACK
1 cup decaffeinated green tea
1 tangerine

LUNCH
2 slices whole-wheat bread topped with
2½ ounces tuna (in water)
1 slice low-fat cheese
3 slices tomato
2 lettuce leaves
2 tablespoons soy mayonnaise
½ cup red grapes
Spring water

AFTERNOON SNACK
1 apple

DINNER
1 Garlicky Turkey Burger*
1 cup steamed cauliflower
½ cup baby carrots
Spring water

Veg Out! *Try our Rice, Corn, and Bean Medley with Cilantro, Coriander, and Cumin for a vegetarian alternative to the turkey burger.*

NIGHTTIME SNACK
½ cup nonfat frozen yogurt
2 tablespoons pecans

Nutrition information: 1,528 calories, 86.2 grams protein or 22 percent, 180.6 grams carbohydrates or 46 percent, 56.8 grams total fat or 32 percent, 173 milligrams cholesterol, 14.3 grams saturated fat or 8 percent, 2,296 milligrams sodium, 28.5 grams dietary fiber

---

Day 3

BREAKFAST
½ whole-grain bagel topped with
1 teaspoon low-fat cream cheese
½ cup orange juice
½ cup low-fat blueberry yogurt

MIDMORNING SNACK
1 cup decaffeinated green tea
1 kiwi

LUNCH
3 ounces skinless chicken breast
2 cups tossed greens
2 ounces marinated artichoke hearts
5 cherry tomatoes
8 mushrooms
1 cup skim milk
1 whole-wheat roll

AFTERNOON SNACK
2 whole-wheat crackers
2 tablespoons peanut butter

DINNER
Whole-wheat pasta in mushroom sauce (1 cup cooked whole-
    wheat pasta stir-fried with 1 tablespoon olive oil, ½ cup shii-
    take mushrooms, 1 garlic clove, ¼ cup chopped onion, ½ cup
    low-sodium chicken broth, and 6 fresh basil leaves)
Spring water

Veg Out! *You can substitute vegetable broth for the chicken broth and still enjoy this tasty dinner.*

Nighttime Snack
1 ounce peanuts

Nutrition information: 1,502 calories, 79.6 grams protein or 20 percent, 178.4 grams carbohydrates or 45 percent, 61.4 grams total fat or 35 percent, 89 milligrams cholesterol, 10.6 grams saturated fat or 6 percent, 1,105 milligrams sodium, 29.6 dietary fiber

---

Day 4

Breakfast
1 cup shredded wheat cereal
¾ cup skim milk
½ whole-wheat English muffin topped with
1½ tablespoons almond butter
Spring water

Midmorning Snack
1 cup decaffeinated green tea
½ cup blueberries

Lunch
1 cup Minestrone*
¼ cup tabbouleh
1 whole-wheat roll
1 orange
Spring water

AFTERNOON SNACK
½ cup low-fat cottage cheese

DINNER
Mexican shrimp (7 medium shrimp stir-fried in 1 tablespoon
    olive oil, 1 roma tomato, and 1 garlic clove) wrapped in
1 whole-wheat tortilla along with
¼ cup avocado and
½ cup salsa
Spring water

Veg Out! *Try our Southwestern Bean Salad for a veggie alternative.*

NIGHTTIME SNACK
1 ounce mixed nuts

Nutrition information: 1,520 calories, 64.6 grams protein or 16
percent, 198.8 grams carbohydrates or 50 percent, 61.4 grams total fat
or 34 percent, 83 milligrams cholesterol, 9.4 grams saturated fat or 5
percent, 2,853 milligrams sodium, 30.5 grams dietary fiber

Day 5

BREAKFAST
2 whole-grain frozen waffles topped with
1 tablespoon apple butter
½ cup raspberries
Spring water

MIDMORNING SNACK
1 cup decaffeinated green tea
½ cup low-fat fruit yogurt

LUNCH
1 piece vegetarian lasagna
1 cup mixed greens topped with
1 tablespoon olive oil and
1 tablespoon vinegar
1 cup skim milk
½ cup fresh pineapple

AFTERNOON SNACK
4 ounces pomegranate juice mixed with 4 ounces water

DINNER
4 ounces baked chicken breast (skinless)
3 ounces baked sweet potato
1 cup red and yellow bell peppers (cooked in 2 teaspoons olive oil)
Spring water

Veg Out! *Our Herbed Polenta with Grilled Portobello Mushrooms is a hearty alternative to a meat dish.*

NIGHTTIME SNACK
1 apricot

Nutrition information: 1,501 calories, 73.9 grams protein or 19 percent, 184.4 grams carbohydrates or 47 percent, 57.9 grams total fat or 34 percent, 147 milligrams cholesterol, 16.2 grams saturated fat or 8 percent, 1,795 milligrams sodium, 21.5 grams dietary fiber

---

Day 6

BREAKFAST
1 cup bran cereal with raisins
1 cup skim milk
1 pear
Spring water

MIDMORNING SNACK
1 cup decaffeinated green tea
½ cup vanilla nonfat yogurt

LUNCH
1 cup vegetarian stew
1 cup mixed green salad combined with
4 olives
2 tomato wedges
2 slices red onion
1 tablespoon olive oil and
1 tablespoon vinegar
Spring water

AFTERNOON SNACK
2 tablespoons natural peanut butter
1 Granny Smith apple

DINNER
3 ounces roasted chicken breast (skinless)
¼ cup garbanzo beans
2 cups Swiss chard stir-fried in
1 tablespoon olive oil with
1 chopped scallion

1 clove garlic and
1 tablespoon chopped fresh dill
Spring water

Veg Out! *Enjoy our Shells Stuffed with Ricotta, Spinach, and Artichokes.*

Nighttime Snack
1 ounce cashews

Nutrition information: 1,495 calories, 78.5 grams protein or 20 percent, 176.5 grams carbohydrates or 45 percent, 61.1 grams total fat or 35 percent, 81 milligrams cholesterol, 10.2 grams saturated fat or 6 percent, 2,107 milligrams sodium, 27.7 grams dietary fiber

---

Day 7

Breakfast
1 cup whole-grain cereal
¾ cup skim milk
1 slice whole-wheat toast topped with
2 teaspoons almond butter
Spring water

Midmorning Snack
1 cup decaffeinated green tea

Lunch
2 slices whole-wheat bread topped with
3 ounces turkey breast
1 tablespoon mustard
2 slices fresh tomato and

2 leaves romaine lettuce
1 baked apple with 1 teaspoon brown sugar
Spring water

AFTERNOON SNACK
1 cup strawberries

DINNER
Southwest Chicken (2 ounces roasted dark-meat chicken stir-
fried in 2 tablespoons olive oil, ½ cup red onion, 1 garlic
clove, 1 teaspoon lime juice, 1 tablespoon fresh cilantro, ½
teaspoon cumin, and ½ teaspoon chili powder) wrapped in
1 whole-wheat tortilla with
1 ounce low-fat Monterey Jack cheese
Spring water

Veg Out! *You might enjoy a Middle Eastern feast of Eggplant, Spinach,
and Garbanzo Bean Curry instead.*

NIGHTTIME SNACK
1 cup nonfat frozen yogurt

Nutrition information: 1,516 calories, 72.8 grams protein or 18
percent, 195.5 grams carbohydrates or 49 percent, 57.6 grams total fat
or 33 percent, 114 milligrams cholesterol, 12.3 grams saturated fat or 7
percent, 2,416 milligrams sodium, 25 grams dietary fiber

My Meal Plans: 2,000 Calories

These meal plans are suitable for most people who are looking to
maintain a healthy weight. However, your age, metabolism, exercise habits, and other factors also come into play. So, once again,

we emphasize the importance of talking with your registered dietitian to find a plan that's right for you.

Day 1

BREAKFAST
1½ cups old-fashioned oatmeal (cooked)
½ cup raspberries
1 slice whole-wheat toast topped with
1 tablespoon almond butter
Spring water

MIDMORNING SNACK
1 cup decaffeinated green tea
6 ounces low-fat strawberry yogurt

LUNCH
1 cup lentil soup
3 ounces turkey breast
1 whole-wheat roll
1 cup cantaloupe
1 cup skim milk

AFTERNOON SNACK
1 ounce peanuts

DINNER
1 serving Snapper with Thyme, Tomatoes, and Kalamata
  Olives*
1 cup asparagus
1½ cups mixed greens combined with
1 tablespoon slivered almonds
1 tablespoon olive oil and

1 tablespoon vinegar
Spring water

Veg Out! *Have a souper dinner of Minestrone as an alternative.*

NIGHTTIME SNACK
1 tablespoon natural peanut butter
4 whole-wheat crackers

Nutrition information: 1,960 calories, 116.9 grams protein or 23 percent, 214.8 grams carbohydrates or 42 percent, 78.9 grams total fat or 35 percent, 114 milligrams cholesterol, 13.1 grams saturated fat or 6 percent, 3,070 milligrams sodium, 33 grams dietary fiber

---

Day 2

BREAKFAST
Power Shake (1 cup frozen strawberries, 1 cup orange juice, 1 ounce soy or whey protein powder, and 1 banana)

MIDMORNING SNACK
1 cup decaffeinated green tea
½ cup low-fat cottage cheese
1 peach

LUNCH
2 slices whole-wheat bread topped with
3 ounces tuna (in water)
3 slices tomato
2 lettuce leaves and
2 tablespoons soy mayonnaise
½ cup red grapes
Spring water

AFTERNOON SNACK
1 apple

DINNER
1 Garlicky Turkey Burger*
1 sweet potato
2 cups cauliflower and broccoli stir-fried in
1½ tablespoons olive oil
Spring water

Veg Out! *Make it Mexican night with our Black Bean and Vegetable Wraps. Olé!*

NIGHTTIME SNACK
1 cup vanilla low-fat frozen yogurt

Nutrition information: 1,970 calories, 115.3 grams protein or 23 percent, 232 grams carbohydrates or 46 percent, 71.9 grams total fat or 32 percent, 172 milligrams cholesterol, 16.2 grams saturated fat or 7 percent, 2,291 milligrams sodium, 32 grams dietary fiber

---

Day 3

BREAKFAST
½ whole-grain bagel
2 teaspoons low-fat cream cheese
1 cup orange juice
1 cup low-fat blueberry yogurt

MIDMORNING SNACK
1 cup decaffeinated green tea
1 pear

LUNCH

3 ounces skinless chicken breast
2 cups tossed green salad combined with
3 ounces marinated artichoke hearts
5 cherry tomatoes
8 mushrooms and
1 tablespoon oil and vinegar dressing
½ cup skim milk
1 whole-wheat roll
Spring water

AFTERNOON SNACK

2 whole-wheat crackers
1 ounce part-skim mozzarella string cheese

DINNER

1 serving Mustard Baked Salmon with Lentils*
½ cup brown rice
1 cup broccoli stir-fried in
1 tablespoon olive oil
Spring water

Veg Out! *Try our quintessential cold soup—Gazpacho topped with a dollop of guacamole—served with our Spinach and Grapefruit Salad as an alternative.*

NIGHTTIME SNACK

1 ounce peanuts

Nutrition information: 2,040 calories, 104.6 grams protein or 20 percent, 238.5 grams carbohydrates or 45 percent, 83.2 grams total fat or 35 percent, 152 milligrams cholesterol, 14.1 grams saturated fat or 6 percent, 2,055 milligrams sodium, 39.5 grams dietary fiber

Day 4

BREAKFAST
1 cup shredded wheat
¾ cup skim milk
1 slice whole-wheat toast topped with
1½ tablespoons natural peanut butter
Spring water

MIDMORNING SNACK
1 cup decaffeinated green tea
1 tangerine

LUNCH
1½ cups Minestrone*
½ cup tabbouleh
¼ cup avocado
1 whole-wheat roll
1 orange
1 cup skim milk

AFTERNOON SNACK
2 cups popcorn cooked in canola oil

DINNER
1 serving Potato and Turkey Hash*
1 cup string beans
1 cup spinach salad combined with
2 radishes
¼ cup celery
¼ cup cucumber
1 tablespoon olive oil and
1 tablespoon vinegar
Spring water

Veg Out! *Our Shells Stuffed with Ricotta, Spinach, and Artichokes put a healthy twist on an old pasta favorite.*

NIGHTTIME SNACK
2 sticks (1 ounce each) part-skim mozzarella string cheese
2 whole-wheat crackers
1 apple

Nutrition information: 1,992 calories, 81.4 grams protein or 16 percent, 279.7 grams carbohydrates or 54 percent, 70.5 grams total fat or 31 percent, 31.4 milligrams cholesterol, 12.8 grams saturated fat or 6 percent, 2,995 milligrams sodium, 42.7 grams dietary fiber

Day 5

BREAKFAST
1 whole-wheat frozen waffle topped with
1 tablespoon natural peanut butter
½ cup blueberries
Spring water

MIDMORNING SNACK
1 cup decaffeinated green tea
2 tangerines

LUNCH
1 serving vegetarian lasagna
1 cup mixed greens combined with
1 tablespoon sesame seeds,
1 tablespoon vinegar, and
½ tablespoon olive oil
1 slice whole-grain bread

1 cup skim milk
½ cup fresh pineapple

Afternoon Snack
1 ounce walnuts

Dinner
4 ounces skinless chicken breast
1 baked sweet potato
1 cup brussels sprouts
1 cup red and yellow bell peppers stir-fried in
1 tablespoon olive oil
1 cup skim milk

Veg Out! *Try our Tabbouleh Primavera paired up with our Chopped Mediterranean Salad.*

Nighttime Snack
½ cup dried apricots
1 cup decaffeinated green tea

Nutrition information: 1,930 calories, 98.6 grams protein or 20 percent, 225.5 grams carbohydrates or 46 percent, 75.9 grams total fat or 35 percent, 186.5 milligrams cholesterol, 18 grams saturated fat or 8 percent, 2,007 milligrams sodium, 30.8 grams dietary fiber

Day 6

Breakfast
1 cup bran cereal with raisins
1 cup skim milk
1 pear
1 cup low-fat vanilla yogurt

MIDMORNING SNACK
1 cup decaffeinated green tea
½ cup low-fat cottage cheese

LUNCH
1 cup vegetarian stew
1 cup mixed green salad combined with
5 green olives
4 tomato wedges
2 slices red onion
1 tablespoon olive oil and
1 tablespoon vinegar
Spring water

AFTERNOON SNACK
1 tablespoon natural peanut butter
1 apple

DINNER
1 serving Shrimp and Broccolini Stir-Fry*
1 cup brown rice
1 cup zucchini stir-fried in
1 tablespoon olive oil
Spring water

Veg Out! *Try our Eggplant, Spinach, and Garbanzo Bean Curry served with whole-wheat pita and cucumber yogurt dipping sauce for a Middle Eastern delight.*

NIGHTTIME SNACK
1 ounce almonds

Nutrition information: 2,041 calories, 109.4 grams protein or 21 percent, 236.1 grams carbohydrates or 45 percent, 81 grams total fat or 35 percent, 282 milligrams cholesterol, 12.7 grams saturated fat or 5 percent, 2,975 milligrams sodium, 33.1 grams dietary fiber

---

Day 7

BREAKFAST
1 cup whole-grain cereal
¾ cup skim milk
½ cup orange juice
1 slice whole-grain toast topped with
1 tablespoon almond butter

MIDMORNING SNACK
1 cup decaffeinated green tea
½ cup strawberries

LUNCH
2 slices whole-wheat bread topped with
3 ounces turkey breast
2 teaspoons mustard
4 slices fresh tomato and
2 leaves romaine lettuce
1 apple
Spring water

AFTERNOON SNACK
1 ounce natural trail mix

DINNER
1 serving Spanish Rice and Chicken Casserole*
2 cups baby spinach combined with
½ cup carrots
¼ cup shredded beets
6 mushrooms
1 ounce toasted sunflower seeds
½ tablespoon olive oil and
1 tablespoon vinegar
Spring water

Veg Out! *Try our Black Bean and Vegetable Wraps served with a mixed green salad as an alternative.*

NIGHTTIME SNACK
½ cup nonfat frozen yogurt
3 tablespoons chopped almonds

Nutrition information: 2,028 calories, 101.9 grams protein or 19 percent, 256.2 grams carbohydrates or 48 percent, 75.6 grams total fat or 32 percent, 131 milligrams cholesterol, 11.2 grams saturated fat or 5 percent, 2,278 milligrams sodium, 37.5 grams dietary fiber

---

My Meal Plans: 2,500 Calories

Some of us may require more calories, either because of a fast metabolism, weight loss from illness and/or treatment, or level of physical activity. Discuss with your health care provider whether the following plan may be right for you.

Day 1

BREAKFAST
1 cup old-fashioned oatmeal (cooked)
½ cup raspberries
1 poached egg
1 slice whole-wheat toast topped with
1 tablespoon almond butter

MIDMORNING SNACK
1 cup decaffeinated green tea
1 apple
½ cup low-fat cottage cheese

LUNCH
1½ cups lentil soup
1 whole-wheat roll topped with
2 ounces chicken breast and
1 tablespoon soy mayonnaise
3 tomato wedges with
2 leaves romaine
1 cup cantaloupe
1 cup skim milk

AFTERNOON SNACK
1 cup low-fat berry yogurt
1 banana

DINNER
1 serving Snapper with Thyme, Tomatoes, and Kalamata
    Olives*
1 cup roasted asparagus with
1 tablespoon olive oil
1 cup whole-wheat pasta

1½ cups mixed greens combined with
1 tablespoon olive oil and
1 tablespoon vinegar
1 slice whole-grain bread

Veg Out! *Go Italian with our Angel-Hair Arrabiata and garlic bread made with whole-grain bread, fresh pressed garlic, and extra-virgin olive oil.*

NIGHTTIME SNACK
6 whole-rye crackers topped with
2 tablespoons natural peanut butter

Nutrition information: 2,517 calories, 132 grams protein or 20 percent, 328 grams carbohydrates or 50 percent, 87 grams total fat or 30 percent, 315 milligrams cholesterol, 13.8 grams saturated fat or 5 percent, 2,093 milligrams sodium, 51.2 grams dietary fiber

---

Day 2

BREAKFAST
Power Shake (1 cup frozen strawberries, 1 cup soy milk, ½ cup low-fat yogurt, 1 ounce soy or whey protein powder, and 1 banana)

MIDMORNING SNACK
1 cup decaffeinated green tea
2 ounces natural trail mix

LUNCH
2 slices whole-wheat bread topped with
⅓ cup egg salad
3 slices tomato and

2 lettuce leaves
½ cup green grapes
1 ounce soy chips

AFTERNOON SNACK
1 orange
1½ ounces peanuts

DINNER
1 Turkey Enchilada*
1 cup sweet potato fries (baked, diced, sautéed)
1 cup steamed cauliflower
Spring water

Veg Out! *Have breakfast for dinner and get a spectrum of phytonutrients with a double serving of our Pumpkin Buckwheat Flapjacks and a Blueberry Mango Soy Smoothie.*

NIGHTTIME SNACK
Fruit salad (½ cup kiwi, ½ cup pineapple, ½ cup mandarin
orange sections, ¼ cup blueberries, and ½ cup vanilla nonfat
frozen yogurt)

Nutrition information: 2,514 calories, 138 grams protein or 21 percent,
323 grams carbohydrates or 48 percent, 92.8 grams total fat or 31
percent, 267 milligrams cholesterol, 20.7 grams saturated fat or 7
percent, 2,908 milligrams sodium, 56.1 grams dietary fiber

Day 3

BREAKFAST
1 whole-grain bagel
1 tablespoon low-fat cream cheese

2 ounces lox
1 cup orange juice

MIDMORNING SNACK
1 cup decaffeinated green tea
½ cup low-fat blueberry yogurt

LUNCH
3 ounces chicken breast
1 baked sweet potato skin
2 cups mixed greens combined with
¼ cup sliced water chestnuts
5 cherry tomatoes and
8 mushrooms
1 cup skim milk
1 whole-wheat roll

AFTERNOON SNACK
1 ounce oil-roasted sunflower seeds
1 cup watermelon
½ whole-wheat English muffin topped with
1 tablespoon almond butter

DINNER
1 serving Mustard Baked Salmon with Lentils*
1 cup brown rice
1 cup broccoli stir-fried in
1 tablespoon olive oil
Spring water

Veg Out! *Try our Black Bean and Vegetable Wraps paired with Emerald Fruit Salad instead.*

NIGHTTIME SNACK
1 ounce mixed nuts
1 apple

Nutrition information: 2,499 calories, 125.8 grams protein or 19 percent, 305 grams carbohydrates or 47 percent, 99.3 grams total fat or 34 percent, 153 milligrams cholesterol, 15.7 grams saturated fat or 5 percent, 2,970 milligrams sodium, 51.4 grams dietary fiber

---

Day 4

BREAKFAST
1 cup shredded wheat
1 cup skim milk
2 tablespoons raisins
1 soft-boiled egg
1 slice whole-wheat toast
Spring water

MIDMORNING SNACK
1 cup decaffeinated green tea
½ cup raspberries

LUNCH
1 cup Minestrone*
½ cup tabbouleh
¼ cup avocado
1 cup red grapes
1 whole-wheat roll
Spring water

AFTERNOON SNACK
½ ounce pecans
1 cup low-fat yogurt

DINNER
1 serving Moroccan Chicken*
1 cup string beans
1 cup spinach salad combined with
2 radishes
5 cherry tomatoes
¼ cup celery
¼ cup cucumber slices
1 tablespoon olive oil and
1 tablespoon vinegar
Spring water

Veg Out! *Shells Stuffed with Ricotta, Spinach, and Artichokes and our Chopped Mediterranean Salad make a perfect pair.*

NIGHTTIME SNACK
4 whole-wheat crackers topped with
2 tablespoons natural peanut butter
8 baby carrots

Nutrition information: 2,498 calories, 112.3 grams protein or 17 percent, 330 grams carbohydrates or 51 percent, 91.1 grams total fat or 32 percent, 371 milligrams cholesterol, 18.2 grams saturated fat or 6 percent, 2,530 milligrams sodium, 44.1 grams dietary fiber

---

Day 5

BREAKFAST
1 whole-wheat waffle topped with
¼ cup maple syrup
1 orange
Spring water

MIDMORNING SNACK
1 cup decaffeinated green tea
1 ounce walnuts
½ cup melon

LUNCH
1 serving vegetarian lasagna
1 cup mixed greens combined with
2 tablespoons sesame seeds
2 teaspoons olive oil and
1 tablespoon vinegar
1 slice whole-grain bread
1 cup skim milk

AFTERNOON SNACK
10 whole-grain corn tortilla chips
½ cup salsa
½ cup black beans
¼ cup low-fat shredded cheese

DINNER
1 serving Shiitake-and-Rappini-Stuffed Chicken Breasts*
1 cup brown rice
½ cup red and yellow bell peppers stir-fried in
1 tablespoon olive oil
Spring water

Veg Out! *Let your blender make your main course tonight. Have our Super Protein Smoothie and a fruit salad.*

Nighttime Snack
⅓ cup dried apricots
¾ cup nonfat frozen yogurt
1 cup decaffeinated green tea

Nutrition information: 2,556 calories, 108.7 grams protein or 17 percent, 342 grams carbohydrates or 52 percent, 90.7 grams total fat or 31 percent, 223 milligrams cholesterol, 22.5 grams saturated fat or 8 percent, 2,835 milligrams sodium, 35.4 grams dietary fiber

---

Day 6

Breakfast
1 cup bran cereal with raisins
1 cup skim milk
1 slice whole-grain toast topped with
2 tablespoons natural peanut butter
1 banana

Midmorning Snack
1 cup decaffeinated green tea
1 cup low-fat blueberry yogurt

Lunch
1 whole-wheat tortilla topped with
⅓ cup hummus and
½ cup grilled tofu
1 cup mixed green salad combined with
4 grilled red pepper strips

2 slices red onion and
1 tablespoon olive oil
1 Granny Smith apple
Spring water

Afternoon Snack
1 cup strawberries
½ cup low-fat cottage cheese

Dinner
1 serving Shrimp and Broccolini Stir-Fry*
1 cup brown rice
1 cup mixed vegetables stir-fried in
1 tablespoon olive oil
Spring water

Veg Out! *Have a double serving of our Black Bean and Vegetable Wraps.*

Nighttime Snack
1 ounce cashews
2 pieces low-fat string cheese

Nutrition information: 2,453 calories, 122.9 grams protein or 19 percent, 295 grams carbohydrates or 46 percent, 99.1 grams total fat or 35 percent, 310 milligrams cholesterol, 20.8 grams saturated fat or 7 percent, 2,483 milligrams sodium, 36.8 grams dietary fiber

---

Day 7

Breakfast
1 cup whole-grain cereal
1 cup skim milk

1 vegetable omelet (½ cup Egg Beaters, ¼ cup green bell
  pepper, and 1 tablespoon canola oil)
½ whole-wheat English muffin topped with
1 tablespoon almond butter
1 cup orange juice

MIDMORNING SNACK
1 cup decaffeinated green tea
1 piece low-fat string cheese
1 pear

LUNCH
2 slices whole-wheat bread topped with
4 ounces turkey (baked deli slices)
2 teaspoons mustard
4 slices fresh tomato and
2 leaves romaine lettuce
1 baked apple topped with
1 teaspoon brown sugar
Spring water

AFTERNOON SNACK
¾ cup raw veggies (carrots, cucumber, cherry tomatoes, pepper
  strips, broccoli)
¼ cup hummus
1 slice toasted whole-wheat bread

DINNER
1 serving Spanish Rice and Chicken Casserole*
1 cup baby spinach combined with
½ cup carrots
¼ cup shredded beets
6 mushrooms
1 tablespoon olive oil and

1 tablespoon vinegar
Spring water

Veg Out! *Have our Minestrone tonight with a mixed green salad.*

NIGHTTIME SNACK
1 cup low-fat vanilla yogurt
½ cup blueberries
1 ounce walnuts

Nutrition information: 2,477 calories, 132.2 grams protein or 21 percent, 311.4 grams carbohydrates or 48 percent, 88.8 grams total fat or 31 percent, 159 milligrams cholesterol, 15.8 grams saturated fat or 6 percent, 3,010 milligrams sodium, 42.5 grams dietary fiber

---

9

Gourmet Rx:
The Recipes

THIS CHAPTER PROVIDES fifty recipes to whet your appetite. You'll find soups and salads, fish and seafood, chicken and turkey, garden entrées, and delicious drinks and desserts. All of these recipes are filled with phytonutrients and will help you toward getting your daily seven to nine servings of fruits and vegetables. In addition, you'll find recipes for smoothies that can help ease symptoms from cancer treatment. Please note that optional ingredients are not included in the nutritional information. Bon appétit!

Soups and Salads

No longer revered as side items, soups and salads take a starring role in your health. Fresh vegetables and a variety of beans help protect your cells from oxidative damage.

Triple Crucifer Soup

This soup is teeming with phytonutrients and makes a perfect accompaniment to a fish dish. For a heartier soup, add tomatoes, kidney beans, white beans, or tofu chunks.

> 2 cups vegetable broth
> ½ cup chopped Vidalia onion
> 2 garlic cloves, crushed
> 1 cup cauliflower florets
> 1 cup broccoli florets
> 2 carrots, sliced
> 1 cup shredded cabbage
> 1 tablespoon mustard seeds
> Freshly ground black pepper

In a medium saucepan, bring the vegetable broth to a boil. Add the onion and garlic, and simmer for 10 minutes. Add the cauliflower, broccoli, carrots, cabbage, and mustard seeds. Grind in black pepper to taste, simmer 20 minutes, and serve.

Makes 4 one-cup servings

Servings of fruits and vegetables: 2 vegetables; **phytonutrients:** indoles, sulforaphane, allicin, sulfides, carotenoids, kaempferol, quercetin

Nutrition information: 73 calories, 3 grams protein, 1 gram total fat, less than 1 gram saturated fat, no cholesterol, 13 grams carbohydrates, 4 grams dietary fiber, 258 milligrams sodium

Chopped Mediterranean Salad

This fresh salad makes liberal use of the cancer-fighting staples in the Mediterranean diet—including olive oil, herbs, and tomatoes. Sautéed shrimp or grilled salmon would be a nice addition to this colorful, crunchy salad.

2 medium tomatoes, seeded and chopped
1 small green bell pepper, seeded and chopped
½ cucumber, seeded and chopped
2 scallions, white and green, chopped
2 tablespoons chopped fresh mint (optional)
1½ tablespoons flat-leaf parsley, chopped
1 tablespoon fresh lemon juice
1 teaspoon extra-virgin olive oil
Salt
Freshly ground black pepper

In a bowl, combine the tomatoes, bell pepper, cucumber, scallions, mint, and parsley. Add the lemon juice and oil. Toss to blend. Season to taste with salt and pepper, and serve.

Makes 4 one-cup servings.

Servings of fruits and vegetables: 1 vegetable; **phytonutrients:** lycopene, sulfides, lignans, flavonoids

Nutrition information: 40 calories, 1 gram protein, 2 grams total fat, less than 1 gram saturated fat, no cholesterol, 7 grams carbohydrates, 2 grams dietary fiber, 11 milligrams sodium

*M*inestrone

There are many varieties of this traditional Italian soup. Ours includes lots of phytoestrogen-rich beans and whole-grain pasta in addition to the colorful combination of vegetables.

1 cup dry kidney beans
1 cup cannellini beans
1 cup peas
4 cloves garlic, sliced
1 large onion, diced
1 28-ounce can crushed tomatoes
2 large carrots, sliced
1 cup broccoli florets
Fresh basil, to taste
Fresh oregano
½ cup small whole-grain pasta
Freshly ground black pepper, if desired

Bring 6 cups of water to a boil in a large pot. Add the kidney beans, cannellini beans, and peas. Add two garlic cloves (sliced) and half the diced onion. Simmer 1 hour (beans should be firm and intact). Add the tomatoes, carrots, broccoli, remaining onion and garlic, basil, and oregano. Simmer over medium-low heat for 20 minutes. Add the pasta, cook 10 minutes, remove from heat, season with pepper if desired, and serve.

Makes 4 one-cup servings.

Servings of fruits and vegetables: 2 vegetables; **phytonutrients:** ferulic acid, indoles, isothiocyanates, phytoestrogens, lycopene, sulfides, carotenoids, allicin

---

Nutrition information: 445 calories, 29 grams protein, 1 gram total fat, less than 1 gram saturated fat, no cholesterol, 84 grams carbohydrates, 25 grams dietary fiber, 74 milligrams sodium

---

Spinach and Grapefruit Salad

Pairing citrus and spinach with crunchy jicama gives an exotic flair to this simple salad. If jicama is not available, substitute water chestnuts.

  1 tablespoon Dijon mustard
  ¼ cup frozen grapefruit juice concentrate
  Sea salt to taste
  Freshly ground black pepper to taste
  2 tablespoons canola oil
  1 yellow grapefruit
  8 cups stemmed flat-leaf spinach, rinsed and dried
  1 cup jicama, cut in ¼-inch cubes

In a small bowl, whisk the mustard and grapefruit juice concentrate with the salt and pepper. Gradually whisk in the oil until the mixture thickens to the consistency of stirred yogurt. Whisk in 3 tablespoons of cold water. Use immediately or store refrigerated in a tightly covered container up to three days. Shake the dressing well before using.

Slice the top and bottom off the grapefruit. With a small, sharp knife, cut away the peel and pith. Holding the grapefruit over a bowl to catch the juices, slip the knife vertically down each side of the individual sections to separate them. Squeeze out any juice from the remaining membrane and add it to the fruit. (Cut sections can be refrigerated in their juice up to two days, tightly covered.)

In a large bowl, toss the spinach with 2 tablespoons of dressing to coat the leaves. Divide the spinach among 4 salad plates. Arrange one-fourth of the grapefruit over the spinach. Sprinkle with one-fourth of the jicama. Drizzle each salad with one-fourth of the remaining dressing. Serve immediately.

Makes 4 one-cup servings.

Servings of fruits and vegetables: 1 fruit, 2 vegetables;
phytonutrients: lutein, zeaxanthin, hesperetin, carotenoids

Nutrition information: 140 calories, 4 grams protein, 8 grams total fat, less than 1 gram saturated fat, no cholesterol, 17 grams carbohydrates, 8 grams dietary fiber, 186 milligrams sodium

---

*E*merald Fruit Salad

A delicious example of "getting your green."

> 2 tablespoons lime juice
> 2 tablespoons clear honey
> 2 green apples, cored and sliced
> 1 small, ripe honeydew melon, diced
> 2 kiwi, sliced
> 1 star fruit, sliced
> Mint sprigs for garnish
> Yogurt to serve

Mix together the lime juice and honey in a large bowl, then toss in the apple slices. Stir in the melon, kiwi, and star fruit. Place in a glass serving dish and chill. Decorate the fruit salad with mint sprigs, and serve with yogurt or fromage frais.

Makes 4 one-cup servings.

Servings of fruits and vegetables: 3 fruit; **phytonutrients:** lutein, zeaxanthin, quercetin

Nutrition information: 170 calories, 2 grams protein, less than 1 gram total fat, no saturated fat, no cholesterol, 45 grams carbohydrates, 6 grams dietary fiber, 48 milligrams sodium

Orange, Watercress, and Red Onion Salad

Three cancer-fighting families—citrus, crucifer, and allium—team up for a light, palate-pleasing salad.

¼ cup extra-virgin olive oil or grapeseed oil
¼ cup orange juice
1 teaspoon orange zest
1 tablespoon balsamic vinegar
1 tablespoon red wine vinegar
2 bunches watercress
4 oranges peeled, pith removed, cut into rounds
1 red onion, sliced
Freshly ground black pepper to taste

Whisk the first five ingredients together. Arrange the watercress, oranges, and onion on a salad plate, and top with vinaigrette and freshly ground black pepper.

Makes 4 one-cup servings.

Servings of fruits and vegetables: 1 fruit, 1 vegetable; **phytonutrients:** hesperetin, isothiocyanates, quercetin, beta-cryptoxanthin

Nutrition information: 216 calories, 2 grams protein, 14 grams total fat, 2 grams saturated fat, no cholesterol, 26 grams carbohydrates, 8 grams dietary fiber, 3 milligrams sodium

Roasted Sweet Potato Soup with Chipotle Pepper Cream

This creamy, comforting soup is chock-full of carotenoids. Pair it with a mixed green salad and some crusty whole-grain bread for a delicious meal.

4 medium sweet potatoes
1 tablespoon olive oil
1 large onion, chopped
½ can chipotle pepper, chopped
1 leek, chopped
4 garlic cloves
9 cups vegetable or free-range chicken stock
½ cup dry white wine
2 teaspoons fresh thyme
½ cup low-fat sour cream
1 teaspoon adobo sauce, made from chipotle peppers

Preheat the oven to 400°F. Prick the potatoes and roast until very tender, about 1¼ hours. Peel and place in a medium bowl. Heat the olive oil in a large pot and sauté the onion until golden, about 8 minutes. Add the sweet potatoes, chipotle pepper, leek, garlic, and 8 cups of the stock. Simmer 20 minutes. Add the wine and thyme, and cook 5 minutes longer. Combine the sour cream and adobo sauce in a small bowl. Puree the soup mixture in batches and transfer to a clean pot. Simmer and add the additional stock to thin, as needed. Ladle the soup into individual bowls, and top with a dollop of the sour cream mixture.

Makes 4 one-cup servings.

Servings of fruits and vegetables: 2 vegetables; **phytonutrients:**
carotenoids, lycopene

Nutrition information: 287 calories, 5 grams protein, 9 grams total fat,
3 grams saturated fat, 12 milligrams cholesterol, 46 grams
carbohydrates, 6 grams dietary fiber, 968 milligrams sodium (This
recipe is high in sodium. Try to reduce your sodium from other sources
to ensure that your total day's intake is moderate.)

Southwestern Bean Salad

A flavorful blend of Latin flavors and full of protein, this salad delivers a delicious dose of phytonutrients.

>   2 15-ounce cans pinto, black, or small white beans, rinsed
>   and drained
>   ½ cup diced red onion
>   ½ cup shredded carrot
>   ½ cup chopped fresh cilantro leaves
>   1 teaspoon cumin
>   2 tablespoons fresh lime juice
>   2 teaspoons extra-virgin olive oil
>   2 teaspoons minced fresh jalapeño or other chili pepper

In a large bowl, combine the beans, onion, carrot, and
cilantro until well mixed. In a small, nonstick skillet, heat the
cumin over low heat just until warm, about 30 seconds. Stir in
the lime juice, oil, and minced jalapeño until blended. Pour the
dressing over the bean salad and toss to blend. Divide evenly
among four salad bowls, and serve.

Makes 4 one-cup servings.

Servings of fruits and vegetables: 1 vegetable; **phytonutrients:** phytoestrogens, quercetin, sulfides, carotenoids

Nutrition information: 222 calories, 11 grams protein, 4 grams total fat, less than 1 gram saturated fat, no cholesterol, 37 grams carbohydrates, 11 grams dietary fiber, 632 milligrams sodium (This recipe is high in sodium. Try to reduce your sodium from other sources to ensure that your total day's intake is moderate.)

Gazpacho

This famous cold soup, which is enjoyed in tropical climates on hot days, is a refreshing treat anytime.

　　6 large ripe tomatoes
　　2 red or yellow bell peppers
　　2 medium yellow onions
　　2 large shallots
　　2 large cucumbers
　　½ cup red wine vinegar or balsamic vinegar
　　⅓ cup extra-virgin olive oil
　　1½ cups tomato juice or V8
　　Juice of 1 lemon
　　1 16-ounce can chickpeas

　　Wash and prepare the vegetables. Core and finely chop the tomatoes; save the juice. Core, seed, and finely chop the peppers, onions, and shallots. Peel the cucumbers and slice them into quarters. In a bowl, whisk together the vinegar, olive oil, reserved tomato juice, canned tomato juice, and lemon. Place all the ingredients in a nonreactive (nonmetal) bowl. Cover and chill for at least 4 hours.

Makes 4 one-cup servings.

Servings of fruits and vegetables: 6 vegetables; **phytonutrients:** lycopene, quercetin, sulfides, phytoestrogens

Nutrition information: 414 calories, 9 grams protein, 21 grams total fat, 3 grams saturated fat, no cholesterol, 53 grams carbohydrates, 10 grams dietary fiber, 99 milligrams sodium

---

Crisp Asian Salad

With a bounty of colorful vegetables from the Orient, this crunchy salad pairs well with our Wasabi Salmon and Edamame.

 12 snow pea pods
 16 yellow or green beans
 1 large carrot, halved and cut in 3-inch-by-¼-inch pieces
 2 cups cut bok choy, white part only
 1 small can water chestnuts, drained
 ¼ cup (about ½ ounce) chives, cut in 2-inch lengths and
    diagonally in ½-inch slices
 2 tablespoons rice vinegar
 2 tablespoons soy sauce
 1 tablespoon fresh lemon juice
 1 teaspoon roasted sesame oil
 ½ teaspoon peanut oil

Bring a medium-sized pot of water to a boil. Fill a large bowl with cold water and ice cubes. Blanch the pea pods for 30 seconds. Use a slotted spoon to transfer them to the ice water. Add the beans to the pot and cook 2 minutes. Transfer them to the ice water. Blanch the carrot pieces 3 minutes; then add them to the ice water. Drain the vegetables well, and place them in a bowl. Add the bok choy, water chestnuts, and chives to the other vegetables. Whisk the vinegar, soy sauce, and lemon juice into the sesame and peanut oils. Pour this dressing over the vegetables, tossing to coat them. Serve immediately.

Makes 4 one-cup servings.

Servings of fruits and vegetables: 2 vegetables; **phytonutrients:** phytoestrogens, isothiocyanates, indoles, sulfides, carotenoids

---

Nutrition information: 66 calories, 2 grams protein, 2 grams total fat, less than 1 gram saturated fat, no cholesterol, 11 grams carbohydrates, 4 grams dietary fiber, 303 milligrams sodium

---

Fish and Seafood

Deep-sea protection!

Steamed Mussels with Saffron Sauce

A spicy dish full of protein with Mediterranean appeal, mussels deliver a good dose of vitamin B$_{12}$ and immune-boosting zinc.

    2 cups fish stock or clam juice
    1 pound mussels, debearded
    1 large onion, chopped
    1 cup dry white wine
    ¼ teaspoon saffron, powdered
    1 tablespoon Dijon mustard
    2 cloves garlic, minced
    ¼ cup extra-virgin olive oil
    4 tablespoons fresh parsley

Simmer fish stock, mussels, onion, and white wine in a saucepan for 15 minutes. Whisk the saffron, mustard, and garlic with the oil. Thin the mixture with 1 tablespoon of fish stock. Bring the rest of the stock to a boil, and stir in 2 tablespoons of the mustard sauce. Cook 5 minutes, until shells open. Divide between 4 bowls, top with parsley, drizzle with remaining mustard sauce over each, and serve.

Makes 4 four-ounce servings.

Servings of fruits and vegetables: 0

Nutrition information: 294 calories, 17 grams protein, 18 grams total fat, 3 grams saturated fat, 33 milligrams cholesterol, 7 grams carbohydrates, less than 1 gram dietary fiber, 610 milligrams sodium (This recipe is high in sodium. Try to reduce your sodium from other sources to ensure that your total day's intake is moderate.)

---

*W*asabi Salmon and Edamame

Omega-3–rich salmon and phytoestrogen-packed soybeans make a perfect combination.

1½ cups sushi rice
2 cups shelled frozen edamame
2 tablespoons reduced-sodium soy sauce
1 tablespoon rice vinegar
1 tablespoon wasabi powder
¼ teaspoon roasted sesame oil
11 ounces salmon, cooked and flaked to yield 1¾ cups
Freshly ground black pepper
4 teaspoons sesame seeds

Rinse the rice in cold water until the water runs clear. Drain well. In a medium saucepan, boil 2 cups plus 2 tablespoons of cold water. Add the rice. When the water returns to a boil, cover the pan and cook 20 minutes without removing the cover. Remove from the heat and let the rice sit 10 minutes, covered, before using.

Boil the edamame in salted water for 4 minutes. Drain and set aside. Whisk together the soy sauce, vinegar, wasabi powder, and oil with 2 tablespoons of water. Set aside. Set a medium, non-stick skillet over medium-high heat. Combine the sauce, salmon, and edamame in the skillet. Warm gently until the fish is completely heated through, about 4 minutes. Season to taste with pepper. Remove the pan from the heat. Divide the cooked rice among 4 plates. Spoon a quarter of the salmon/edamame mixture, including sauce, over the rice. Sprinkle the sesame seeds on top and serve.

Makes 4 five-ounce servings.

Servings of fruits and vegetables: 1 vegetable; **phytonutrients:** phytoestrogens, isoflavones

Nutrition information: 284 calories, 22 grams protein, 7 grams total fat, less than 1 gram saturated fat, 14 milligrams cholesterol, 31 grams carbohydrates, 5 grams dietary fiber, 765 milligrams sodium (This recipe is high in sodium. Try to reduce your sodium from other sources to ensure that your total day's intake is moderate.)

Mustard Baked Salmon with Lentils

This hearty Mediterranean-inspired meal pairs lentils with fish for a dish that's full of protein and fiber, not to mention a boatload of phytonutrients.

    2 cups lentils
    1 cup diced carrots
    ½ cup diced celery
    1 cup chopped leeks
    ½ cup chopped onion

6 whole garlic cloves
1 bay leaf
⅓ cup olive oil
2 tablespoons white wine vinegar
¼ cup large-grain mustard
4 3-ounce salmon fillets
½ cup chopped parsley

Rinse the lentils and combine them with the carrots, celery, leeks, onion, garlic, bay leaf, and 3 tablespoons of the olive oil in a pot. Sauté over medium heat for 5 minutes. Add 4 cups of water and cover. Simmer 1 hour until tender. Turn off the heat, and add the vinegar. Preheat the oven to 425°F. Blend the mustard and remaining olive oil, and spread the mixture onto the 4 salmon fillets. Oil a cooking rack and place it in a roasting pan. Place the fillets on the rack and cook 10 minutes. Stir the parsley into the lentil mixture and divide it among 4 plates. Place the salmon atop the lentils and serve.

Makes 4 four-ounce servings.

Servings of fruits and vegetables: 2 vegetables; **phytonutrients:** quercetin, sulfides, kaempferol, carotenoids, lignans, phytoestrogens

Nutrition information: 466 calories, 28 grams protein, 26 grams total fat, 4 grams saturated fat, 447 milligrams cholesterol, 32 grams carbohydrates, 11 grams dietary fiber, 688 milligrams sodium (This recipe is high in sodium. Try to reduce your sodium from other sources to ensure that your total day's intake is moderate.)

Crispy Citrus Tuna

The combination of citrus and tuna gives this omega-3–rich dish a lot of zing. Serve with steamed bok choy or broccoli to round out a delicious Asian meal.

  2 large oranges
  1½ cups orange juice
  2 tablespoons dry white wine (optional)
  2 tablespoons cornstarch or arrowroot
  2 tablespoons chopped fresh cilantro
  2 tablespoons cornmeal
  ½ teaspoon sea salt (optional)
  ¼ teaspoon black pepper
  4 6-ounce tuna steaks, ½ inch thick
  4 teaspoons olive oil

Peel and section the oranges. Whisk the orange juice, wine (if desired), and cornstarch or arrowroot in a small saucepan until smooth. Bring to a boil over medium-high heat and cook, stirring constantly, until sauce boils and thickens, about 2 minutes. Remove from the heat and stir in the orange sections. Keep warm. Mix the cilantro, cornmeal, salt, and pepper in a pie plate. Coat both sides of the tuna steaks with the cornmeal mixture, pressing firmly so the mixture adheres. Heat 2 teaspoons of the oil in a large, cast-iron skillet over medium-high heat until hot but not smoking. Sear the tuna until done to taste, 2 to 3 minutes on each side for medium-rare. Add the remaining oil just before turning the fish. Serve with the sauce.

Makes 4 six-ounce servings.

Servings of fruits and vegetables: 2 fruit; **phytonutrients:** hesperetin

---

Nutrition information: 349 calories, 42 grams protein, 7 grams total fat, 1 gram saturated fat, 77 milligrams cholesterol, 28 grams carbohydrates, 3 grams dietary fiber, 353 milligrams sodium

---

Fillet of Sole Florentine

A lighter seafood dish, sole provides B vitamins necessary for proper division of cells. Try it with our Orange, Watercress, and Red Onion Salad.

1½ cups spinach, raw
¼ cup dry bread crumbs
1 tablespoon minced shallots
½ teaspoon fresh rosemary or ¼ teaspoon dried and crushed
½ teaspoon fresh thyme leaves or ¼ teaspoon dried
3 to 4 gratings fresh nutmeg, or pinch of ground
¼ teaspoon salt, or to taste
¼ teaspoon fresh ground white pepper, or to taste
1 pound fillet of sole, divided into 4 pieces
½ cup vegetable or chicken broth
1 teaspoon cider vinegar
1 teaspoon sugar
Paprika for garnish

Preheat the oven to 350°F. In a large bowl, mix together the spinach, bread crumbs, shallots, rosemary, thyme, nutmeg, salt, and pepper. Arrange the spinach mixture to cover the bottom of an 8-inch square or other shallow baking dish just large enough to hold the fish in one layer. Arrange the fish over the spinach, overlapping as little as possible. In a small saucepan, combine the broth, vinegar, and sugar and bring just to a boil. Pour the hot liquid over the fish. Dust the fillets lightly with paprika. Bake until the fish is an opaque white all the way through. Serve immediately.

Makes 4 four-ounce servings.

Servings of fruits and vegetables: 0

Nutrition information: 141 calories, 23 grams protein, 2 grams total fat, less than 1 gram saturated fat, 55 milligrams cholesterol, 7 grams carbohydrates, less than 1 gram dietary fiber, 221 milligrams sodium

---

Grilled Grouper with Cilantro Cantaloupe Salsa

The cilantro-based salsa adds a nice bite to the mild grouper, which delivers a healthy dose of B vitamins. Serve it with black beans and brown rice.

> Juice and zest of 1 lemon
> ½ cantaloupe, diced
> ⅓ cup finely chopped cilantro
> 1 shallot, diced
> 2 grouper fillets
> Freshly ground black pepper
> Vegetable oil spray

Combine the lemon juice and zest, cantaloupe, cilantro, and shallot in a glass bowl. Rinse the fish and lightly coat with oil (spray). Cover the fish with one-third of the salsa, making sure not to contaminate the salsa with fish juice. Refrigerate the fish to marinate, 20 minutes to 2 hours. Prepare the grill and cook the fish approximately 10 minutes per side, or until it is white and flaky in the center. Top with the remaining salsa and black pepper, and serve.

Makes 4 four-ounce servings.

Servings of fruits and vegetables: 1 fruit; **phytonutrients:** carotenoids

Nutrition information: 163 calories, 25 grams protein, 5 grams total fat, less than 1 gram saturated fat, 48 milligrams cholesterol, 4 grams carbohydrates, less than 1 gram dietary fiber, 73 milligrams sodium

---

Shrimp and Broccolini Stir-Fry

Asian inspiration! The ginger and hot pepper in this fast and healthy stir-fry give this meal spicy appeal.

- 2 tablespoons canola oil
- 1½ pounds large shrimp (about 30), peeled and deveined
- 3 teaspoons grated, peeled fresh ginger
- 4 teaspoons minced garlic
- 2 bunches (8 ounces) broccolini or broccoli rabe, cut into ¼-inch-thick diagonal slices
- 3 tablespoons hoisin sauce
- 3 tablespoons reduced-sodium soy sauce
- ½ teaspoon dried hot red pepper flakes

Heat 1 tablespoon of the oil in a large, nonstick skillet over moderately high heat until hot but not smoking. Cook the shrimp until golden and almost cooked through, about 1 minute on each side, and then transfer to a dish. Heat the remaining tablespoon of oil in the skillet over moderately high heat until hot but not smoking, then sauté the ginger and garlic, stirring until golden. Add the broccolini, 1 cup water, hoisin, soy sauce, and red pepper flakes. Cook, stirring occasionally, just until the broccolini is tender, about 5 minutes. Stir in the shrimp and cook until heated through. Serve with brown rice.

Makes 4 servings of seven shrimp each.

Servings of fruits and vegetables: 1 vegetable; **phytonutrients:** gingerols, indoles, isothiocyanates

Nutrition information: 309 calories, 38 grams protein, 11 grams total fat, 1 gram saturated fat, 259 milligrams cholesterol, 14 grams carbohydrates, less than 1 gram dietary fiber, 857 milligrams sodium (This recipe is high in sodium. Try to reduce your sodium from other sources to ensure that your total day's intake is moderate.)

Snapper with Thyme, Tomatoes, and Kalamata Olives

This snapper is a snap to make and absolutely delicious. You can find Kalamata olives in the prepared foods cooler of your grocery store.

6 large plum tomatoes, coarsely chopped
2 shallots, chopped
4 teaspoons chopped fresh thyme
2 tablespoons extra-virgin olive oil

4 6- to 7-ounce red or yellowtail snapper fillets
10 Kalamata olives, halved

Combine the plum tomatoes, shallots, and chopped thyme in a small bowl. Cut two sheets of aluminum foil about 18 inches long and place them on the work surface. Drizzle ½ tablespoon of the olive oil in the center of each piece of foil. Place two snapper fillets side by side in the center of each piece of foil. Top with the tomato mixture, and sprinkle with olives. Drizzle the fish with the remaining tablespoon of olive oil. Fold the foil over each packet, enclosing the contents completely and crimping the edges to seal tightly. (This can be prepared up to 6 hours ahead and refrigerated.)

Preheat the oven to 450°F. Place a large baking sheet in the oven and heat 10 minutes. Place the foil packets on the heated baking sheet. Bake until the fish is opaque in the center, about 15 minutes. Remove from the oven; let stand 5 minutes. Serve over brown rice.

Makes 4 six-ounce servings.

Servings of fruits and vegetables: 3 vegetables; **phytonutrients:** lycopene, sulfides, quercetin

---

Nutrition information: 320 calories, 38 grams protein, 12 grams total fat, 2 grams saturated fat, 63 milligrams cholesterol, 15 grams carbohydrates, 1 gram dietary fiber, 270 milligrams sodium

Sea Bass Provençale

Sea bass is a hearty, firm-fleshed fish that's especially rich in B vitamins. Pair it with our Chopped Mediterranean Salad.

¼ cup chopped oil-packed sun-dried tomatoes, drained
    with 2 tablespoons oil reserved
1 tablespoon drained capers
1 tablespoon chopped garlic
1 tablespoon minced fresh basil or 1½ teaspoons dried
½ cup dry white wine
½ cup bottled clam juice
4 6-to 7-ounce sea bass fillets

Preheat the oven to 450°F. Heat the 2 tablespoons of reserved oil in a large, heavy, ovenproof skillet over medium-high heat. Add the tomatoes, capers, garlic, and basil, and stir 1 minute. Add the wine and clam juice, and boil until the liquid is reduced almost to a glaze, about 3 minutes. Add the fish to the skillet; turn to coat with the sauce. Place the skillet in the oven. Roast the fish until it is just opaque in the center, about 15 minutes. Transfer the fish and sauce to a platter.

Makes 4 six-ounce servings.

Servings of fruits and vegetables: 1 vegetable; **phytonutrients:**
sulfides, lycopene

Nutrition information: 204 calories, 32 grams protein, 4 grams total fat, 1 gram saturated fat, 71 milligrams cholesterol, 3 grams carbohydrates, less than 1 gram dietary fiber, 264 milligrams sodium

Citrus-Soy Scallops with Soba Noodles

Soba noodles are made from buckwheat and can be found in the Asian section of your grocery store or at a health-food store.

¼ cup reduced-sodium soy sauce
¼ cup fresh lemon juice
¼ cup fresh lime juice
2 teaspoons finely grated, peeled fresh ginger
2 teaspoons sesame oil
1 8-ounce package soba (buckwheat) noodles
2 pounds large sea scallops (about 30), tough muscle
removed from side of each if necessary
2 teaspoons vegetable oil

Whisk together the soy sauce, lemon and lime juices, ginger, and sesame oil in a wide, shallow, nonreactive bowl. Boil water for the soba noodles, add the noodles, and cook until al dente. Meanwhile, add the scallops to the lemon-soy mixture and marinate, covered, at room temperature, for 5 minutes on each side. (Do not marinate longer or the scallops will become mushy when they're cooked.) Transfer the scallops to a plate and reserve the marinade. Heat ½ teaspoon vegetable oil in a 12-inch nonstick skillet over moderately high heat until hot but not smoking. Then sauté the scallops, six to eight at a time, until golden brown and just cooked through, 2 to 3 minutes on each of the flat sides, transferring them to a plate as they're cooked. Wipe out the skillet and add ½ teaspoon oil between batches. Wipe out the skillet again, then add the marinade, and boil until reduced to about ⅓ cup, about 2 minutes. Place the scallops over the soba noodles, and drizzle with sauce.

Makes 4 eight-ounce servings.

Servings of fruits and vegetables: 0

Nutrition information: 448 calories, 47 grams protein, 7 grams total fat, less than 1 gram saturated fat, 75 milligrams cholesterol, 52 grams carbohydrates, less than 1 gram dietary fiber, 1,348 milligrams sodium (This recipe is high in sodium. Try to reduce sodium from other sources to ensure that your total day's intake is moderate.)

Chicken and Turkey

Poultry provides a bevy of B vitamins.

Double Veggie Chicken Soup

The quintessential comfort food.

1¾ cups free-range chicken broth
1 pound skinless, boneless, free-range chicken breasts
1 medium onion, chopped
2 tablespoons olive oil
1 garlic clove, minced
4 medium carrots, cut diagonally into ⅓-inch-thick slices
2 celery ribs, cut crosswise into ⅓-inch-thick slices
1 cup sliced bok choy, green and white parts
1 teaspoon salt
¼ teaspoon black pepper
3 tablespoons finely chopped fresh parsley
½ cup celery leaves

Bring 4 cups of water and broth to a simmer in a large saucepan. Add the chicken and simmer, uncovered, 6 minutes. Remove the pan from the heat and cover; let stand until the chicken is cooked through, about 15 minutes. Transfer the chicken to a plate and cool 10 minutes. Reserve the poaching liquid, uncovered. While the chicken is poaching, cook the onion in oil in a covered 4-quart heavy pot, over moderate heat, stirring occasionally, until softened but not browned, about 6 minutes. Add the garlic and cook, stirring occasionally, until fragrant, about 1 minute. Add the carrots, celery, bok choy, salt, and pepper, and cook, covered, stirring occasionally, until softened, 8 to 10 minutes. Add the poaching liquid and simmer, covered, until the vegetables are tender, about 10 minutes. Remove from the heat. While the vegetables are cooking, shred the chicken into ¼-inch-wide strips (about 1 inch long). When the vegetables are done simmering, stir the chicken into the soup along with the parsley and celery leaves.

Makes 4 ten-ounce servings.

Servings of fruits and vegetables: 1 vegetable; **phytonutrients:** quercetin, lignans, sulfides, carotenoids, isothiocyanates, indoles

Nutrition information: 247 calories, 29 grams protein, 9 grams total fat, 2 grams saturated fat, 68 milligrams cholesterol, 11 grams carbohydrates, 3 grams dietary fiber, 161 milligrams sodium

Shiitake-and-Rappini-Stuffed Chicken Breasts

Stuffed with health! The mushrooms and broccoli rabe add powerful phytonutrients to this mouthwatering meal.

1 tablespoon extra-virgin olive oil or canola oil
1 shallot peeled, minced
1 pound shiitake mushrooms, stems removed, chopped
2 cloves garlic
Freshly ground black pepper
3 cups broccoli rabe (rappini), finely chopped
⅓ cup finely chopped parsley
2 boneless, skinless, free-range chicken breasts, split
    (4 pieces)

Heat oven to 400°F. In a large skillet, warm the oil over medium heat. Add the shallot, stirring with a wooden spoon for 1 minute. Add the mushrooms and garlic, stirring about 4 minutes. Season with black pepper, add the broccoli rabe over mushrooms, cover, and steam 2 minutes. Remove from the heat, add the parsley, and mix well. Slice a 3-inch section of the chicken horizontally to form a pocket. Spoon in ⅓ cup of the mushroom filling into each of the breasts, tuck the ends under, and secure them with a toothpick. Place the chicken in a roasting pan, spray with olive oil, and season with black pepper. Bake to a golden brown, about 35 minutes, and serve.

Makes 4 five-ounce (stuffed) servings.

Servings of fruits and vegetables: 2 vegetables; **phytonutrients:** lentinan, lignans, sulfides, isothiocyanates, indoles

Nutrition information: 223 calories, 31 grams protein, 5 grams total fat, less than 1 gram saturated fat, 66 milligrams cholesterol, 11 grams carbohydrates, 2 grams dietary fiber, 117 milligrams sodium

Chicken Piperade

This simple chicken and vegetable medley is quick to prepare. We suggest serving it over brown rice.

½ tablespoon extra-virgin olive oil
2 large red bell peppers, seeded and cut into ½-inch strips
2 large yellow bell peppers, seeded and cut into ½-inch strips
1 medium Spanish onion, halved and cut crosswise

1 garlic clove, minced
¾ pound boneless, skinless, free-range chicken breast
1 teaspoon sea salt
Freshly ground pepper

Heat the oil in a deep, medium skillet over medium-high heat. Add the peppers, onion, and garlic. The pan will be heaped with the vegetables. Sauté, stirring often, until the peppers have softened and the red ones have become lighter in color, about 10 minutes. The pan will be moist from the juices of the peppers. Add the chicken and stir until the pieces are white all over. Cook, stirring occasionally, until the peppers and onions are very soft and lightly browned in places, 20 to 25 minutes. The chicken should be white all the way through and tender. Season to taste with salt and pepper.

Makes 4 four-ounce servings.

Servings of fruits and vegetables: 3 vegetables; **phytonutrients:** sulfides, allicin, quercetin, lycopene, lignans

Nutrition information: 173 calories, 22 grams protein, 3 grams total fat, less than 1 gram saturated fat, 49 milligrams cholesterol, 15 grams carbohydrates, 3 grams dietary fiber, 636 milligrams sodium

Oven-Baked Chicken Fingers

A healthy twist on a homestyle favorite, choose this better-for-you alternative when a fried chicken urge strikes.

2 teaspoons canola oil
½ teaspoon sea salt
⅛ teaspoon freshly ground black pepper
Pinch cayenne pepper
1 cup rolled oats (not quick-cooking)
1 large egg white
About ¾ pound boneless, skinless chicken breasts (preferable free-range)
½ cup honey mustard
2 tablespoons low-fat yogurt
2 tablespoons reduced-fat sour cream

Place a rack in the center of the oven. Preheat the oven to 450°F. Coat a baking sheet with cooking spray and set aside. In a medium bowl, whisk together the oil, salt, pepper, and cayenne. Place the oats in a blender and process until they're coarsely ground. Add the oatmeal to the oil mixture and work it with your fingers until the oil is well distributed. Transfer the mixture to a flat plate. In another bowl, whisk the egg white until foamy. Cut the chicken lengthwise into 5½-inch strips. Dip the chicken in the egg white, then roll in the oat mixture, pressing with your fingers to help it adhere. Arrange the coated chicken slices on the prepared baking sheet. Coat them generously with cooking spray. Bake until the chicken is tender when pierced with a wooden pick and the coating is golden and crisp, about 15 minutes. Cool 5 minutes on the baking sheet.

Meanwhile, in a small bowl, mix together the mustard, yogurt, and sour cream. Place the bowl in the center of a serving plate. Arrange the chicken fingers around the dip, and serve.

Makes 4 three-ounce servings.

Servings of fruits and vegetables: 0

Nutrition information: 354 calories, 25 grams protein, 16 grams total fat, 2 grams saturated fat, 53 milligrams cholesterol, 29 grams carbohydrates, 2 grams dietary fiber, 440 milligrams sodium

Moroccan Chicken

This chicken dish is warmed with fragrant spices and served with couscous. Try the unique flavor combination when you're in the mood for something a little different.

¼ teaspoon ground turmeric or saffron threads
2 tablespoons extra-virgin olive oil
1 large onion, chopped fine
2 1½-pound skinless, free-range chicken breasts (total)
2½ pounds ripe plum tomatoes, peeled, seeded, and
   chopped
1 teaspoon ground cinnamon
1 teaspoon ground ginger
3 tablespoons honey (preferably wildflower)
1 teaspoon sea salt
4 cups cooked hot couscous

If using saffron, place it in a small bowl and add 2 table-spoons of hot water. Let it sit until saffron is dissolved, about 20 minutes, before using. Heat the oil in a large, deep pan over medium-high heat. Sauté the onion until golden, about 6 minutes. Remove with a slotted spoon and transfer to a plate. Add the chicken and sauté, turning frequently, until browned on all sides, about 8 minutes. Remove the chicken to plate with the onion and set aside. Pour ½ cup water into the pan, scraping the bottom with a wooden spoon to loosen all the browned bits. Add the tomatoes and cook until softened, about 8 minutes. Stir in the turmeric (or saffron), cinnamon, ginger, honey, and salt to taste. Return the chicken and onion to the pan. Cover tightly and simmer gently until the chicken is very tender, about 50 minutes. Serve ladled over hot couscous.

Makes 4 six-ounce servings.

Servings of fruits and vegetables: 1 vegetable; **phytonutrients:** curcumin, quercetin, sulfides, gingerols, lycopene

---

Nutrition information: 657 calories, 44 grams protein, 24 grams total fat, 6 grams saturated fat, 109 milligrams cholesterol, 67 grams carbohydrates, 6 grams dietary fiber, 718 milligrams sodium (This recipe is high in sodium. Try to reduce your sodium from other sources to ensure that your total day's intake is moderate.)

Spanish Rice and Chicken Casserole

A comforting casserole with a health conscience, this complete meal includes peppers, tomatoes, peas, brown rice, and onions to complement the chicken.

1¼ cups long-grain brown rice
1 medium onion, chopped

1 tablespoon extra-virgin olive oil

1 14½-ounce can stewed tomatoes

1¼ cup free-range chicken broth, divided

1 teaspoon paprika

½ teaspoon dried oregano

½ teaspoon freshly ground black pepper

1 7-ounce jar roasted red peppers, drained and chopped

2 medium (about 1¼ pounds total), skinless, boneless, free-range chicken breasts

1 bay leaf

½ cup frozen green peas

Sea salt to taste

Freshly ground black pepper to taste

Preheat the oven to 375°F. In a 2-quart casserole, combine the rice, onion, and oil. Mix in the tomatoes, 1 cup of the broth, paprika, oregano, ground pepper, roasted peppers, chicken, and bay leaf. Cover the casserole and bake 30 minutes. Stir in the peas and add an additional ¼ cup broth, if needed to keep rice from sticking. Bake until the rice is tender and the chicken is cooked through, about 20 minutes. Remove the bay leaf, add salt and pepper, if desired, and serve.

Makes 4 four-ounce servings.

Servings of fruits and vegetables: 3 vegetables; **phytonutrients:** ferulic acid, lycopene, lignans, isoflavones, quercetin, sulfides

Nutrition information: 510 calories, 42 grams protein, 9 grams total fat, 2 grams saturated fat, 83 milligrams cholesterol, 68 grams carbohydrates, 7 grams dietary fiber, 561 milligrams sodium

*P*otato and Turkey Hash

A quick, Southern-style jumble, our Potato and Turkey Hash can be served as a hearty breakfast.

> 2 large potatoes, sliced thin (about 3 cups)
> 1 large onion, chopped
> 1 cup diced turkey (preferably free range)
> ⅓ cup diced mixed red and green bell peppers
> 1½ teaspoons Worcestershire sauce
> 1 teaspoon minced garlic
> 2 scallions, chopped
> 1 tablespoon olive oil
> 1 to 2 dashes hot pepper sauce, or to taste
> Sea salt and freshly ground black pepper to taste

In a large, nonstick skillet, bring the potatoes, 1½ cups water, and onion to a boil. Cover and cook over medium heat for 10 minutes, or until the vegetables are tender. Drain and return the vegetables to the pan. Add the turkey, bell peppers, Worcestershire sauce, garlic, scallions, oil, and hot pepper sauce. Mix well. Cook, uncovered, over medium heat for about 5 minutes, stirring occasionally, until the mixture begins to brown. Season with sea salt and black pepper to taste.

Makes 4 four-ounce servings.

Servings of fruits and vegetables: 1 vegetable; **phytonutrients:** quercetin, lignans, sulfides, allicin, lycopene

Nutrition information: 224 calories, 9 grams protein, 5 grams total fat, less than 1 gram saturated fat, 12 milligrams cholesterol, 37 grams carbohydrates, 4 grams dietary fiber, 247 milligrams sodium

Grilled Chicken Packets

This no-mess meal is full of herbs and spices that enhance the flavors of the chicken and vegetables.

1 Spanish onion, cut into ½-inch slices
1 large Granny Smith apple, peeled, quartered, and diced
1 large green bell pepper, seeded and cut into ½-inch slices
12 ounces skinless, boneless, free-range chicken breast, cut into strips
1 cup "lite" coconut milk
4 teaspoons curry powder
2 teaspoons finely minced fresh ginger
¼ cup chopped fresh cilantro
Salt and freshly ground black pepper to taste

Heat an outdoor grill or preheat the oven to 400°F. Lay out 4 10-inch-long sheets of heavy-duty, wide foil. Place one-fourth of the onion slices in the center of each piece of foil. Cut each apple quarter into 4 slices and arrange over the onion. Lay one-fourth of the pepper strips over the apple. Cut each chicken piece into 4 strips. Arrange over the peppers. In a small bowl, combine the coconut milk, curry powder, ginger, cilantro, and salt and pepper to taste. Pour a quarter of the mixture over the chicken and vegetables in each packet. Bring the sides of the foil together and roll them down over the center of each packet. Roll each end in to seal. Place the packets on the grill, cover the grill, and cook until the chicken is cooked through, about 15 minutes. (Or set the packets on a baking sheet and bake until the chicken is done, about 20 minutes.)

Makes 4 three-ounce servings (over rice).

Servings of fruits and vegetables: 1 fruit, 1 vegetable; **phytonutrients:** quercetin, gingerols, ferulic acid, curcumin

Nutrition information: 470 calories, 27 grams protein, 15 grams total fat, 11 grams saturated fat, 49 milligrams cholesterol, 58 grams carbohydrates, 7 grams dietary fiber, 76 milligrams sodium

Turkey Enchiladas

Mexican food can be healthy! We leave out the sneaky "bad" fats found in most Mexican dishes but keep the phytoestrogen-rich beans. Be sure to read the labels on tortillas to make sure no hydrogenated oils are present.

1½ cups diced cooked turkey (preferably free range)
1 15-ounce can pinto beans, rinsed and drained
1 14¾-ounce can creamed corn
⅔ cup reduced-fat sour cream, or dairy-free soy sour cream
3 scallions, green and white parts, chopped
6 corn tortillas (nonhydrogenated)
½ cup green salsa
Dairy-free soy cheddar cheese slices

Preheat the oven to 375°F. Combine the turkey and beans in a bowl. Mix the corn, ½ cup of the sour cream, and scallions together in another bowl. Soften and warm the tortillas by placing them, one at a time, directly on a gas burner grid over a medium flame, until warm and flat, 20 to 30 seconds, turning once. Repeat until all the tortillas are warm. (If using an electric stove, use a dry, cast-iron skillet over medium heat. Place one tortilla at a time in the skillet and heat on both sides, about 45 seconds in total.) To keep tortillas warm during this process, stack them on a plate and cover with a dish towel.

Spread half the salsa over the bottom of an 8-inch square baking dish. Cover with two tortillas, tearing the second one in half to fit. Spread half the turkey mixture over the tortillas. Cover with half the corn mixture. Lay four slices of cheese over the corn. Add another layer of tortillas. Cover with the remaining salsa, turkey, and corn mixtures. Lay the rest of the tortillas on top. Spread the remaining sour cream over the tortillas. Top with the remaining cheese. Bake uncovered until the casserole is bubbly and heated through, 25 to 30 minutes. Let stand 10 minutes before serving.

Makes 4 three-ounce servings.

Servings of fruits and vegetables: 1 vegetable; **phytonutrients:** isoflavones, quercetin, zeaxanthin

---

Nutrition information: 552 calories, 42 grams protein, 21 grams total fat, 8 grams saturated fat, 59 milligrams cholesterol, 60 grams carbohydrates, 11 grams dietary fiber, 1,077 milligrams sodium (This recipe is high in sodium. Try to reduce sodium from other sources to ensure that your total day's intake is moderate.)

Garlicky Turkey Burgers

In the mood for a burger? Try this beef alternative and serve with roasted sweet potato wedges.

　　1 pound ground free-range turkey breast
　　½ cup whole-wheat bread crumbs

1 10-ounce package frozen chopped spinach, thawed
1 cup chopped onion
6 tablespoons Dijon mustard, divided
Pinch of sea salt
¼ cup sliced, roasted red peppers
4 ounces part-skim mozzarella cheese, cut into 4 slices

In a large bowl, thoroughly combine the turkey, bread crumbs, spinach, onion, 4 tablespoons mustard, and salt. Shape the mixture into 4 patties. Cover them with plastic wrap and chill 30 minutes. Grill the burgers or sauté them in a nonstick skillet over medium heat for 8 to 10 minutes on each side, or just until the turkey is firm and no longer pink. (Do not overcook.) When the burgers are almost completely cooked, spread the top of each with 1½ teaspoons mustard and 1 tablespoon red peppers, then top each with a slice of cheese. Continue cooking just until the cheese begins to melt. (Cover so the cheese will melt easily.) Serve immediately on whole-grain buns.

Makes 4 four-ounce servings.

Servings of fruits and vegetables: 1 vegetable; **phytonutrients:** quercetin, lutein, zeaxanthin, lycopene

Nutrition information: 351 calories, 31 grams protein, 17 grams total fat, 6 grams saturated fat, 105 milligrams cholesterol, 16 grams carbohydrates, 3 grams dietary fiber, 1,035 milligrams sodium (This recipe is high in sodium. Try to reduce sodium from other sources to ensure that your total day's intake is moderate.)

Garden Entrées

On the lighter side, these meals are a perfect example of how to give your vegetables center stage without sacrificing flavor.

Tabbouleh Primavera

A Middle Eastern favorite, tabbouleh brings you cancer-fighting grains and greens. It can also be found in the deli section of your grocery store.

1 cup bulgur wheat
1 pound thin asparagus, cut into ½-inch pieces
1 medium bell pepper, diced
2 tablespoons extra-virgin olive oil
4 ounces mixed bean sprouts
4 scallions, sliced thin
2 medium carrots, shredded
2 medium tomatoes, diced
3 tablespoons fresh lemon juice
⅓ cup chopped flat-leaf parsley
2 tablespoons chopped mint
2 cups mixed greens, or 1 head Boston lettuce

Boil 2½ cups water over high heat; stir in the bulgur. Reduce the heat to low, cover, and simmer 15 minutes. Drain and let cool. In a medium skillet, combine the asparagus and ½ cup water. Cover and simmer over high heat for 2 minutes. Drain and return to the burner, add the pepper and 1 tablespoon oil. Cook about 2 minutes over medium-high heat. Combine the asparagus mixture with the bulgur and 1 tablespoon oil. Add all other ingredients except the greens. Arrange the greens or lettuce on plates, and top with the bulgur mixture.

Makes 4 one-cup servings.

Servings of fruits and vegetables: 3 vegetables; **phytonutrients:** ferulic acid, glutathione, lycopene, lignans, sulfides, carotenoids, lycopene, lutein, zeaxanthin

---

Nutrition information: 266 calories, 9 grams protein, 8 grams total fat, 1 gram saturated fat, no cholesterol, 43 grams carbohydrates, 12 grams dietary fiber, 36 milligrams sodium

---

*M*editerranean Gateau

Layers of protection! This layered vegetable dish is full of phytonutrients and is a meal on its own.

⅓ cup olive oil, plus oil to grease
1 medium eggplant, cut into ¼-inch slices
2 tablespoons chopped fresh basil or cilantro
1 garlic clove
4 bell peppers (2 red, 1 yellow, and 1 green), roasted and
    peeled
4 plum tomatoes, cut into thick slices
2 tablespoons red wine vinegar
6 tablespoons olive oil
Salt to taste
Freshly ground black pepper
Fresh basil sprig for garnish

Preheat the oven to 350°F. Heat ¼ cup of the olive oil in a heavy-bottomed skillet. Cook the eggplant for 5 minutes on each side over medium heat until golden. Drain. In a blender or food processor, puree together the basil and garlic with 2 tablespoons of olive oil. Place four 3-inch metal ring molds on a lightly greased baking sheet. Layer the vegetables in the molds: start with a slice of eggplant, then continue with 1 teaspoon of basil puree; alternate pieces of the red, yellow, and green peppers; more basil puree; another slice of eggplant; and then basil puree again. Top with a layer of tomatoes. Press down lightly, drizzle with the remaining olive oil, and then bake for 10 minutes. Place the molds on serving plates; then carefully lift off the molds. Blend together all the remaining ingredients for the vinaigrette. To serve, garnish each gateau with a drizzle of vinaigrette and a sprig of basil.

Makes 4.

Servings of fruits and vegetables: 5 vegetables; **phytonutrients:** lignans, anthocyanins, sulfides, lycopene

---

Nutrition information: 451 calories, 4 grams protein, 40 grams total fat, 6 grams saturated fat, no cholesterol, 22 grams carbohydrates, 7 grams dietary fiber, 16 milligrams sodium

---

Herbed Polenta with Grilled Portobello Mushrooms

Polenta, a cooked cornmeal product, has been enjoyed since Roman times. Ours teams up with hearty portobellos for a delicious meatless meal.

2 teaspoons extra-virgin olive oil
1 cup noninstant polenta or cornmeal
1 small garlic clove, minced
¼ cup chopped flat-leaf parsley
1 teaspoon crumbled fresh thyme leaves, or ¼ teaspoon dried
1 teaspoon finely chopped fresh rosemary, or ¼ teaspoon dried
Salt
Freshly ground black pepper, to taste
¼ cup (1 ounce) grated parmigiano-reggiano cheese
4 large portobello mushrooms, stems removed

Preheat the oven to 350°F. In a deep, heavy pot, combine the oil and polenta. Cook over medium-high heat, stirring, until the polenta smells toasty, about 2 minutes. Remove the pot from heat. Add 4 cups of boiling water carefully to avoid spatters. Stir until the polenta is smooth. Mix in the garlic, parsley, thyme, rosemary, salt, and pepper. Bake the polenta, uncovered, 20 minutes. Stir well. Bake an additional 20 minutes, or until the polenta is creamy.

Slice polenta and divide among 4 dinner plates. Sprinkle each with a quarter of the cheese. While the polenta cooks, lightly coat the mushroom caps with canola oil spray, sprinkle with salt, and grill, underside (gills) down, on a very hot grill or in a heavy cast-iron pan, about 4 minutes. Turn and cook until tender all the way through, about 4 minutes. Top each serving of polenta with a mushroom and serve immediately.

Makes 4 four-ounce servings.

Servings of fruits and vegetables: 1 vegetable; **phytonutrients:** zeaxanthin, lignans, sulfides, isoflavones

Nutrition information: 200 calories, 7 grams protein, 5 grams total fat, 1 gram saturated fat, 4 milligrams cholesterol, 32 grams carbohydrates, 4 grams dietary fiber, 101 milligrams sodium

*A*ngel-Hair Arrabiata

Pasta and red sauce get a makeover with whole-wheat angel-hair and red pepper flakes. Delicioso! Healthful hint: Scientists have found that when you let crushed garlic stand, it enhances the formation of health-promoting compounds.

3 cloves of garlic, pressed or chopped
2 tablespoons grapeseed oil or extra-virgin olive oil
8 vine-ripened fresh tomatoes, chopped, or 2 16-ounce
   cans whole tomatoes
¼ cup chopped fresh sweet basil
¼ cup chopped fresh oregano
¼ cup finely chopped fresh parsley
½ teaspoon crushed red pepper
Freshly ground black pepper to taste
Whole-wheat angel-hair pasta
Fresh Parmesan or mozzarella cheese to taste (optional)

Allow the garlic to stand 10 minutes after chopping or pressing. In a medium saucepan, add the oil, and heat to medium-low. Add the tomatoes, garlic, herbs, and red pepper to the oil; grind in black pepper. Simmer over medium-low heat for 20 minutes, stirring with a wooden spoon. The longer the sauce simmers, the richer and spicier the flavor will become. Cook the pasta according to box directions. Drain, spoon the sauce over it, top with cheese if desired, and garnish with additional herbs.

Makes 4 four-ounce servings.

Servings of fruits and vegetables: 1 vegetable; **phytonutrients:** lycopene, sulfides, lignans

---

Nutrition information: 280 calories, 10 grams protein, 8 grams total fat, 1 gram saturated fat, 1 milligram cholesterol, 46 grams carbohydrates, 8 grams dietary fiber, 37 milligrams sodium

---

Shells Stuffed with Ricotta, Spinach, and Artichokes

Traditional stuffed shells get spinach and artichokes tucked in for added flavor and phytonutrients.

1 artichoke, halved and sharp ends trimmed
Juice of 1 lemon
1 tablespoon extra-virgin olive oil, canola oil, or grapeseed oil
2 cups low-fat or fat-free ricotta
3 cloves garlic, crushed
2 16-ounce cans low-sodium whole tomatoes
1 10-ounce box whole-grain large pasta shells
2 cups fresh flat-leaf spinach

½ tablespoon pine nuts (optional)
¼ cup fresh basil for garnish

Preheat the oven to 350°F. In a saucepan, heat 2 cups of water with the halved artichoke, lemon juice, and ½ tablespoon oil. Cover and simmer 35 to 40 minutes. While the artichoke simmers, combine the ricotta and 2 garlic cloves; refrigerate. Place the whole tomatoes and 1 garlic clove in a saucepan over low heat. Cook the pasta according to package directions. Sauté the spinach in a spray of oil, stirring occasionally, 3 minutes. Remove from the heat and transfer the spinach to a cutting board. Chop it well, and add to the ricotta mixture. Drain the artichoke, remove the fuzzy choke, and peel the leaves. Chop the artichoke leaves coarsely. Combine with the ricotta and spinach mixture. Add ½ tablespoon pine nuts if desired. Spoon the mixture into the shells and arrange them in a glass baking dish. Top the shells with the tomatoes and bake for 20 minutes. Garnish with fresh basil, and serve.

Makes 4 six-ounce servings.

Servings of fruits and vegetables: 1.5 vegetables; **phytonutrients:** ferulic acid, lignans, lycopene, sulfides

Nutrition information: 447 calories, 24 grams protein, 14 grams total fat, 7 grams saturated fat, 39 milligrams cholesterol, 57 grams carbohydrates, 5 grams dietary fiber, 214 milligrams sodium

Grilled Fruit Kebabs

Heat up these cool fruits and add some spice for an unusually delicious combination.

2 tablespoons canola oil
2 tablespoons date sugar
2 tablespoons fresh lemon juice
1 teaspoon cinnamon
2 apples, cored and cut into 1-inch pieces
2 bananas, peeled and cut into 1-inch pieces
2 peaches, nectarines, or plums (or a mix), pitted
2 pears, pitted and cut into 1-inch pieces
4 1-inch slices canned or fresh pineapple, cut into quarters

In a small bowl, stir together the oil, date sugar, lemon juice, and cinnamon until the sugar is dissolved. Thread the fruit, alternating types, onto each of 8 skewers. Brush the kebabs with the oil mixture and place the skewers on a barbecue grill. Turn frequently until the fruit starts to brown, about 6 to 8 minutes.

Makes 4 six-ounce servings.

Servings of fruits and vegetables: 3 fruit; **phytonutrients:** quercetin, carotenoids

Nutrition information: 238 calories, 2 grams protein, 4 grams total fat, less than 1 gram saturated fat, no cholesterol, 54 grams carbohydrates, 11 grams dietary fiber, 2 milligrams sodium

Rice, Corn, and Bean Medley with Cilantro, Coriander, and Cumin

A Southwestern combination—rice, corn, and beans—makes a complete protein source that's light and delicious. Ours gets a boost with herbs and spices that create an unforgettable flavor.

2 garlic cloves, minced
1 cup chopped onion
2 teaspoons ground cumin
1 teaspoon ground coriander
½ teaspoon sea salt
1 cup brown rice
1 15-ounce can black beans, rinsed
1 cup corn
6 tablespoons chopped fresh cilantro
2 tablespoons fresh lime juice
Sea salt and freshly ground black pepper
1 red bell pepper, chopped

In a medium saucepan, bring 2 cups of water, garlic, onion, cumin, coriander, and salt to a boil. Stir in the rice, reduce the heat to simmer, cover, and cook about 40 minutes, or until the liquid is absorbed. Transfer the rice to a large bowl to cool. When it is completely cooled, stir in the beans, corn, cilantro, and lime juice. Season to taste with salt and pepper. Transfer to a large serving bowl. Garnish with red bell pepper.

Makes 4 six-ounce servings.

Servings of fruits and vegetables: 1 vegetable; **phytonutrients:** sulfides, isoflavones, zeaxanthin, lycopene

Nutrition information: 276 calories, 10 grams protein, 2 grams total fat, less than 1 gram saturated fat, no cholesterol, 61 grams carbohydrates, 9 grams dietary fiber, 815 milligrams sodium (This recipe is high in sodium. Try to reduce sodium from other sources to ensure that your total day's intake is moderate.)

*P*umpkin Buckwheat Flapjacks

Pancakes on their best behavior! These whole-grain flapjacks get a nutritional boost of carotenoids from the pumpkin.

1 cup buckwheat flour
2 tablespoons packed brown sugar
1½ teaspoons baking powder
½ teaspoon baking soda
1 teaspoon ground cinnamon
1 teaspoon ground ginger
½ teaspoon freshly grated nutmeg
Pinch of cloves
Pinch of salt
1⅓ cups buttermilk
2 large eggs or egg substitute
1 teaspoon pure vanilla extract
¾ cup canned, solid-pack pumpkin

In a medium bowl, whisk together the flour, brown sugar, baking powder, baking soda, spices, and salt. In another bowl, whisk together the buttermilk, eggs, and vanilla to blend thoroughly. Pour the liquid ingredients over the dry ingredients, and mix with the whisk, stopping when everything is just combined.

With a rubber spatula, gently but thoroughly fold in the pumpkin. Spray the griddle or skillet. Preheat over medium heat, or if using an electric griddle, set to 350°F. (If you want to hold the pancakes until serving time, preheat your oven to 200°F.)

Spoon ¼ cup of the batter onto the griddle for each pancake, allowing space for spreading. When the undersides of the pancakes are golden and the tops are lightly speckled with bubbles that pop and stay open, flip the pancakes over with a wide spatula and bake until the other side is light brown. (These pancakes are soft and puffy, so turn carefully.) Serve immediately, or keep cooked pancakes in the preheated oven while you make the rest of the batch. Serve the pancakes hot with a drizzle of honey or pure maple syrup, and chopped nuts or dried fruits, if desired.

Makes 4 four-ounce servings.

Servings of fruits and vegetables: 0; **phytonutrients:** carotenoids, quercetin, gingerols

---

Nutrition information: 196 calories, 8 grams protein, 4 grams total fat, 1 gram saturated fat, 107 milligrams cholesterol, 34 grams carbohydrates, 5 grams dietary fiber, 302 milligrams sodium

---

Eggplant, Spinach, and Garbanzo Bean Curry

This Indian-inspired meal gets its golden hue from the curcumin found in turmeric.

    1 large eggplant with skin, diced
    ½ teaspoon sea salt for sprinkling
    2 tablespoons black mustard seeds

3 tablespoons extra-virgin olive oil or canola oil

1 large onion, diced

1 16-ounce can garbanzo beans, drained and rinsed well

2 bunches spinach, stems removed, washed, and cut into
   2-inch pieces

2 tablespoons minced garlic

2 tablespoons freshly grated ginger

1 teaspoon garam masala (Indian Spice Mix found in
   Chapter 4)

¼ teaspoon turmeric

¼ teaspoon cayenne pepper

2 medium tomatoes, peeled, seeded, and diced

Place the eggplant in a colander, sprinkle with sea salt, and let stand for 30 minutes to sweat. Pat dry with paper towels. Place the mustard seeds in a small, dry sauté pan and cook over moderate heat until they turn gray and start popping. Remove from the heat and reserve. Heat half of the oil in a large skillet over moderate heat. Sauté the eggplant, stirring occasionally, until soft and golden. Remove from the heat and reserve in a bowl with the mustard seeds.

Heat the remaining oil in a medium saucepan over medium-high heat. Add the onion and garbanzo beans. Sauté until the onion is golden and soft. Add the spinach, stirring until wilted, about 2 minutes. Mix in the garlic and ginger, and cook just until aromas are released, then stir in all the spices. Cook an additional minute, stirring constantly to blend spices and prevent scorching. Add the tomatoes and 1 cup of water. Turn the heat to high and bring to a boil, and stir in the eggplant mixture. When the eggplant is heated through, about 2 minutes, remove from the heat and serve.

Makes 4 six-ounce servings.

Servings of fruits and vegetables: 4 vegetables; **phytonutrients:** flavonoids, lutein, zeaxanthin, isoflavones, lignans, quercetin, sulfides, curcumin, lycopene

Nutrition information: 290 calories, 12 grams protein, 13 grams total fat, 2 grams saturated fat, no cholesterol, 38 grams carbohydrates, 14 grams dietary fiber, 442 milligrams sodium

*B*lack Bean and Vegetable Wraps

Health under wraps! Beans, peppers, onions, and zucchini get tucked into a whole-wheat shell to create a flavorful, nutritional standout.

> 1½ tablespoons olive oil
> 2 large garlic cloves, minced
> 1 cup diced red bell pepper
> 1 cup diced yellow bell pepper
> 1 cup ½-inch pieces zucchini
> 1 cup chopped red onion
> 2 teaspoons ground cumin
> 1 15-ounce can black beans, drained
> 1 cup (packed) grated hot-pepper Monterey Jack cheese, or
>   soy pepper jack cheese
> 4 9- to 10-inch-diameter flour tortillas (nonhydrogenated)
> 4 tablespoons chopped fresh cilantro
> Sea salt to taste
> Fresh ground black pepper to taste

Heat the olive oil in a large, heavy skillet over medium-high heat. Add the garlic and stir 30 seconds. Add the bell peppers, zucchini, and onion, and sauté until crisp-tender, about 8 minutes. Mix in the cumin and sauté until the vegetables are tender, about 2 minutes longer. Season with salt and pepper. Place the beans in a large bowl; mash coarsely with a fork. Mix in the vegetables and cheese.

Place the tortillas on a work surface. Spoon one-fourth of the filling down the center of each. Sprinkle each with 1 tablespoon cilantro. Roll up the tortillas, enclosing the filling. Arrange the wraps, seam side down, on a baking sheet. Preheat the oven to 350°F. Cover the wraps with foil. Bake until the filling is just heated through, about 10 minutes. Cut each wrap into 2 or 3 sections.

Makes 4 six-ounce servings.

Servings of fruits and vegetables: 2 vegetables; **phytonutrients:** isoflavones, lycopene, lignans, quercetin

---

Nutrition information: 391 calories, 16 grams protein, 18 grams total fat, 7 grams saturated fat, 25 milligrams cholesterol, 46 grams carbohydrates, 8 grams dietary fiber, 863 milligrams sodium (This recipe is high in sodium. Try to reduce sodium from other sources to ensure that your total day's intake is moderate.)

Desserts and Drinks

Who says dessert can't be healthy? Try these and other nutrition-packed desserts to ease your treatment and please your palate without guilt.

Blueberry Mango Soy Smoothie

Berry delicious! This perfect combination can be enjoyed at breakfast or as an afternoon snack.

½ cup orange juice
1 cup fresh or frozen blueberries
1 cup silken tofu
1 large mango, diced

Place all ingredients in a blender. Blend until smooth.

Makes 2 twelve-ounce servings.

Servings of fruits and vegetables: 2 fruit; **phytonutrients:** anthocyanins, carotenoids, isoflavones, hesperetin

Nutrition information: 204 calories, 7 grams protein, 4 grams total fat, less than 1 gram saturated fat, no cholesterol, 38 grams carbohydrates, 4 grams dietary fiber, 10 milligrams sodium

Banana Berry Cooler

Try different varieties of berries in this delightful mix.

½ cup strawberry sorbet
1 cup cranberry juice
1 cup fresh blueberries
1 frozen banana, sliced

Place all ingredients in a blender. Blend until smooth.

Makes 2 eleven-ounce servings.

Servings of fruits and vegetables: 3 fruit; **phytonutrients:** ellagic acid, anthocyanins

Nutrition information: 230 calories, 1 gram protein, less than 1 gram total fat, less than 1 gram saturated fat, no cholesterol, 57 grams carbohydrates, 4 grams dietary fiber, 22 milligrams sodium

Super Protein Smoothie (Coping Cuisine)

This smoothie is perfect for increasing protein and calories when you're undergoing treatment.

¾ cup almond milk
½ cup plain low-fat yogurt
½ cup silken tofu
⅓ cup (about 8) chopped dates
2 tablespoons peanut butter
1 frozen banana

Place all ingredients in a blender. Blend until smooth.

Makes 1 twenty-two-ounce serving.

Servings of fruits and vegetables: 5 fruit; **phytonutrients:** isoflavones

Nutrition information: 670 calories, 23 grams protein, 23 grams total fat, 4 grams saturated fat, 8 milligrams cholesterol, 103 grams carbohydrates, 10 grams dietary fiber, 221 milligrams sodium

---

Fig and Apricot Compote (Coping Cuisine)

This is a high-fiber dessert or breakfast to keep everything running smoothly.

½ ounce fresh ginger, peeled and sliced thin
¼ teaspoon fennel seeds
2 tea bags (black tea)
6 ounces (about 1 cup) dried apricots, halved
2 ounces dried black figs
2 tablespoons honey
Plain low-fat yogurt

Bring 2 cups of spring water to a boil, then add the ginger and fennel. Add the tea bags and remove from the heat. Let stand 2 minutes. Remove the tea bags. Add the apricots, figs, and honey; return to a boil. Reduce heat and simmer, partially covered, until the liquid is absorbed and the fruit is tender, about 20 minutes. Serve warm or chilled with yogurt on the side, if desired.

Makes 2 fifteen-ounce servings.

Servings of fruits and vegetables: 5 fruit; **phytonutrients:** carotenoids, ferulic acid, flavonoids, anthocyanins, tannins

Nutrition information: 399 calories, 7 grams protein, 1 gram total fat, less than 1 gram saturated fat, 4 milligrams cholesterol, 91 grams carbohydrates, 8 grams dietary fiber, 53 milligrams sodium

Full of Fiber Smoothie (Coping Cuisine)

Increasing your fiber is delicious with this smoothie. You can substitute prunes for the dates if you like.

½ cup plain, low-fat yogurt
⅔ cup buttermilk
⅓ cup dates
2 bananas
2 tablespoons bran
3 to 4 ice cubes

Place all ingredients in a blender. Blend until smooth.

Makes 1 twenty-two-ounce serving.

Servings of fruits and vegetables: 6 fruit; **phytonutrients:** ferulic acid, flavonoids

Nutrition information: 504 calories, 16 grams protein, 5 grams total fat, 3 grams saturated fat, 14 milligrams cholesterol, 113 grams carbohydrates, 13 grams dietary fiber, 298 milligrams sodium

Tummy-Soothing Smoothie (Coping Cuisine)

The ginger in this smoothie helps to ease an upset stomach.

    ¾ cup green tea
    1 cup diced apricots
    ¾ cup papaya
    2 tablespoons pineapple juice
    ¼ teaspoon ginger

Place all ingredients in a blender. Blend until smooth.

Makes 1 sixteen-ounce serving.

Servings of fruits and vegetables: 2 fruit; **phytonutrients:** carotenoids, gingerols, tannins, catechins

Nutrition information: 137 calories, 3 grams protein, less than 1 gram total fat, less than 1 gram saturated fat, no cholesterol, 33 grams carbohydrates, 6 grams dietary fiber, 6 milligrams sodium

Hydrating Smoothie (Coping Cuisine)

A light and refreshing drink.

    2 cups diced, seeded watermelon
    1 cup frozen strawberries
    2 teaspoons lemon juice
    4 ounces Gatorade (try lemon-lime or watermelon)

Place all ingredients in a blender. Blend until smooth.

Makes 2 ten-ounce servings.

Servings of fruits and vegetables: 1 fruit; **phytonutrients:** ellagic acid, lycopene

Nutrition information: 87 calories, 1 gram protein, less than 1 gram total fat, less than 1 gram saturated fat, no cholesterol, 20 grams carbohydrates, 2 grams dietary fiber, 28 milligrams sodium

---

*E*nergizing Smoothie (Coping Cuisine)

Feeling fatigued? Sip on this citrus-and-tea-based smoothie for an energizing boost.

1 cup orange segments, chilled
½ cup grapefruit segments, chilled
½ cup strongly brewed Earl Grey tea, chilled
¾ cup orange sherbet
2 ice cubes, crushed

Combine the orange segments, grapefruit segments, and tea in a blender. Add the sherbet and ice. Blend until smooth.

Makes 2 ten-ounce servings.

Servings of fruits and vegetables: 1 fruit; **phytonutrients:** hesperetin, beta-cryptoxanthin, tannins, catechins

Nutrition information: 136 calories, 2 grams protein, 1 gram total fat, less than 1 gram saturated fat, 3 milligrams cholesterol, 32 grams carbohydrates, 3 grams dietary fiber, 26 milligrams sodium

Frozen Gingered Peach Yogurt Pie

A slice of health! This nourishing version of an American favorite boasts a carotenoid-rich peach filling inside a wheat-germ crust.

¾ cup wheat germ
2 cups graham cracker crumbs (nonhydrogenated)
⅓ cup grapeseed oil
1 32-ounce container plain low-fat yogurt
¼ ounce fresh ginger, grated
6 peaches, diced

In a large bowl, combine the wheat germ, graham cracker crumbs, ⅓ cup of water, and oil. Mix well and press firmly into pie pan, using wax paper. Place the yogurt, ginger, and half of the diced peaches in a blender. Blend on high for 1 minute. Add the remaining peaches (left whole) and pour into the pie shell. Freeze 4 hours.

Makes 8 servings (one-eighth of pie).

Servings of fruits and vegetables: 1 fruit; **phytonutrients:** flavonoids, carotenoids, ferulic acid, gingerols

Nutrition information: 297 calories, 9 grams protein, 13 grams total fat, 2 grams saturated fat, 7 milligrams cholesterol, 37 grams carbohydrates, 3 grams dietary fiber, 207 milligrams sodium

Mocha Soy Pudding

Oh, soy! Here's a healthier version of the grocery-store variety of pudding to quell your chocolate cravings.

2 10½-ounce packages silken tofu
⅔ cup light brown sugar
5 tablespoons cocoa powder
1¼ teaspoons cinnamon
2 teaspoons instant coffee
Mint leaves for garnish

Drain the tofu and pat dry with paper towels. Place it in a food processor with the sugar, cocoa, and cinnamon. In a cup, mix the coffee and 2 teaspoons of boiling water; add to the processor. Process the mixture until smooth, scraping the sides of the container to incorporate all ingredients. Spoon into dessert dishes, top with mint, and chill 30 minutes.

Makes 4 six-ounce servings.

Servings of fruits and vegetables: 0; **phytonutrients:** isoflavones, catechins

Nutrition information: 186 calories, 9 grams protein, 5 grams total fat, less than 1 gram saturated fat, no cholesterol, 32 grams carbohydrates, less than 1 gram dietary fiber, 17 milligrams sodium

10

Help on the Road to Recovery

IT IS NATURAL for anyone who has finished cancer treatment to be concerned about what the future holds. You may be concerned about the way you look and feel. Or you may worry about whether the cancer will return and wonder what you can do to prevent that. Understanding what to expect after cancer treatment can help survivors and their families plan for follow-up care, adjust to necessary lifestyle changes, stay optimistic, and make important decisions. This chapter is dedicated to those readers who are living with cancer and provides information on follow-up care, wellness planning, cancer resources, and support groups.

Staying Well: A Lifelong Process

All cancer survivors should have follow-up care. However, you may have a lot of questions about getting that care:

* Whether to tell the doctor about symptoms that worry you
* Which doctors to see after treatment
* How often to see the doctor
* What specific tests you need and how often

❖ What you can do to relieve pain and other problems after treatment

❖ How long it will take for you to recover from treatment and feel more like yourself

Dealing with these issues can be a challenge, but getting involved in decisions about your future medical care and lifestyle is a good way to regain some of the control you may feel you have lost during treatment. Research has shown that people who feel more in control function better than those who do not. Being an active partner with your doctor and getting help from other members of your health care team is an important step.

The main purpose of follow-up care is to determine whether your cancer has returned (recurrence) or if it has spread to another part of your body (metastasis). Follow-up care can also help in finding other types of cancer and in spotting side effects from treatment that occur immediately or develop years later. At follow-up visits, your doctor will review your medical history and give you a physical exam. Follow-up tests—including imaging procedures (ways of producing pictures of areas inside the body), endoscopy (the use of a thin, lighted tube to examine organs inside the body), and blood tests—are routinely performed to get an accurate picture of your progress.

Changes You May Want to Think About

After cancer treatment, many survivors take a good look at health-promoting activities in their lives to focus on secondary prevention. By developing a wellness plan, you and your health-care team can implement ways to take care of your physical, emotional, and spiritual needs. Making healthy changes in the way you live can help you feel better and may also lower your chances of developing other health problems, such as heart disease or diabetes.

Eating Well After Cancer Treatment

Eat a variety of healthful foods, with an emphasis on foods from plant sources. This means you should try to do the following:

* Eat five or more servings of vegetables and fruits each day.
* Choose whole grains rather than processed (refined) grains and sugars.
* Limit red meats, especially high-fat or processed meats.
* Choose foods that help you maintain a healthy weight.

Exercising After Cancer Treatment

While it may be difficult to do, it's important to be physically active to help maintain a healthy weight after treatment. Studies have shown that moderate exercise (walking, biking, or swimming) for about thirty minutes every—or almost every—day can have several benefits:

* Reducing anxiety and depression
* Improving mood
* Boosting self-esteem
* Reducing symptoms of fatigue, nausea, pain, and constipation from the aftereffects of treatment

During recovery, it is important to start an exercise program slowly and increase your level of activity over time. Work with your health-care team to create a plan that's right for you.

Making Additional Changes

Additional changes you should make, if you haven't already, include quitting smoking and cutting down on how much alcohol you drink. Research shows that smoking can increase the chances of developing cancer at the same or another site. Similarly, drinking alcohol can increase your chances of developing certain cancers.

Resources to Get Started: Commitment to a Cure

Many organizations offer ways to get involved in the fight against cancer. Either through fund-raising events or direct donation, your contribution can make an important impact on the lives of those suffering from cancer and their loved ones.

American Cancer Society

The American Cancer Society (ACS), with more than thirty-four hundred local offices, is committed to fighting cancer through balanced programs of research, education, patient service, advocacy, and rehabilitation. The ACS offers many events and services, including the following:

✣ Relay for Life is an overnight event in local communities across the nation to raise money for cancer. You can walk, run, or just show your support through a donation.

✣ Making Strides Against Breast Cancer raises awareness and dollars to fight this disease. The walks happen nationwide throughout the year and are typically five miles in length.

✣ Coaches vs. Cancer brings together the American Cancer Society and the National Association of Basketball Coaches in the fight against cancer.

Contact Info. phone: 800-ACS-2345, **website:** cancer.org

Susan G. Komen Breast Cancer Foundation

The Susan G. Komen Breast Cancer Foundation supports innovative research and community-based outreach programs in the fight against breast cancer. It was founded by two sisters—Susan Goodman Komen and Nancy Goodman Brinker. Susan was diagnosed with breast cancer in 1978. Before she died at the age of thirty-six, she asked her sister to do everything possible to bring an end to breast cancer. Nancy established the foundation in 1982 in Susan's memory. Working through a network of U.S. and international affiliates and events such as the following, the Komen Foundation is fighting to eradicate breast cancer:

❖ **Race events.** The Komen Race for the Cure® Series is the largest series of five-kilometer runs and fitness walks in the world. The Race celebrated its twenty-first anniversary in 2004, and more than a million people were expected to participate in more than one hundred races around the United States.

❖ **Fund-raising and awareness programs.** The Komen Foundation is a grassroots network consisting of more than seventy-five thousand volunteers worldwide. Affiliates in more than one hundred cities enhance awareness of the disease and raise funds to support a variety of community-based outreach projects and a centralized research initiative.

Komen also offers breast cancer and health education, advocacy and public policy programs, grant-making programs, and survivor programs.

Contact Info. phone: 800-I'M AWARE (800-462-9273), **website:** komen.org

Lance Armstrong Foundation

The Lance Armstrong Foundation was created by cancer survivor and cycling champion Lance Armstrong.

Contact Info. phone: 512-236-8820, **website:** http://laf.org

Super Support: Communities for Cancer

Support groups can have many benefits. You may feel better about yourself, find a new life focus, learn about better pain control, make new friends, improve your mood, cope better with your cancer, learn more about cancer, and deal more effectively with the needs of others in your life. The number-one reason people join a support group is to be with other people who have "been there"—not because they do not receive support from friends and family. Some research shows that joining a specific type of support group improves quality of life and enhances survival.

Numerous types of support groups exist. Some may be for one type of cancer only; others may be open to those with any type of cancer. Some are gender-specific, while others may be focused on people in certain ethnic or racial groups. Support groups may be led by health professionals or fellow cancer survivors.

Support groups are not just for people who have had cancer; they are also helpful for children or family members of survivors. These groups focus on family concerns such as role changes, relationship changes, financial worries, and how to support the person who had cancer. Some groups include both cancer survivors and family members.

Internet support groups can also be a big help to people with computers who live in rural areas or who have trouble getting to meetings. With Internet groups, you can seek support at any time of the day or night. However, while these groups can provide valuable emotional support, they may not always offer correct medical information. Always talk with your doctor before making any changes. Support groups vary greatly, so take the time to find one with which you're comfortable. You may also want to consider finding another cancer survivor with whom you can discuss your experiences. Many organizations can pair you with someone who had your type of cancer and is close to your age and background.

Cancer Survivors Network

This is both a telephone- and Web-based service for cancer survivors, and their families, caregivers, and friends. When you call, the service provides survivors and families access to prerecorded discussions. The Web-based component offers live online chat sessions, virtual support groups, prerecorded talk shows, and personal stories.

Contact Info. phone: 877-333-HOPE (877-333-4673), **website:** http://acscsn.org

Additional General Cancer Resources

Numerous resources exist for dealing with the issues surrounding cancer—from treatment options to emotional issues.

Cancer Information Service

The Cancer Information Service (CIS) is the National Cancer Institute's link to the public, interpreting and explaining research findings in a clear and understandable manner. The CIS can respond to specific questions about cancer, including ways to prevent cancer, how to quit smoking, symptoms and risks, diagnosis, current treatments, and research studies. Whether you use the phone or the Internet, you can contact knowledgeable, caring staff who are trained to explain medical information in terms you can easily understand.

Contact info. phone: 800-4-CANCER (800-422-6237), **TTY:** 800-332-8615; **website:** http://cis.nci.nih.gov (Click on the Live Help link between 9:00 A.M. and 5:00 P.M., Eastern time, Monday through Friday.)

Office of Cancer Survivorship

The National Cancer Institute's Office of Cancer Survivorship provides information on new and innovative research in cancer survivorship and links to information on follow-up medical care after cancer treatment, late effects, health and well-being, and getting involved after cancer treatment.

Contact info. website: http://dccps.nci.nih.gov/ocs

National Cancer Information Center

The American Cancer Society's National Cancer Information Center (NCIC) is a nationwide information service, available twenty-four hours a day, seven days a week to answer calls and e-mails from cancer patients, their families and friends, and individuals. Specially trained cancer information specialists have access to large databases of information and can help answer complex questions regarding diagnoses, side effects, and interactions of treatments. They also have oncology nurse information specialists to assist with other cancer-related questions.

You will be able to speak with a cancer information specialist any day or anytime. Staff can accept calls in either English or Spanish and can distribute publications in both languages.

Contact info. phone: 800-ACS-2345 (800-227-2345)

Look Good . . . Feel Better

In partnership with the Cosmetic, Toiletry, and Fragrance Association Foundation and the National Cosmetology Association, this free program teaches female cancer patients beauty techniques to help restore their appearance and self-image during chemotherapy and radiation treatments.

Contact info. website: http://lookgoodfeelbetter.org

Cancer Care, Inc.

Cancer Care is a national nonprofit agency that offers free support, information, financial assistance, and practical help to people with cancer and their loved ones. Services are provided by oncology social workers and are available in person, over the telephone, or through the agency's website. Cancer Care also provides education, information, and assistance to health care professionals. A section of the Cancer Care website and some publications are available in Spanish, and staff can respond to calls and e-mails in English or Spanish.

Contact info. phone: 800-813-HOPE (800-813-4673), **website:** http://cancercare.org

National Coalition for Cancer Survivorship (NCCS)

This is a network of groups and individuals that offers support to cancer survivors and their loved ones. It provides information and resources on cancer support, advocacy, and quality-of-life issues. A section of the NCCS website and a limited selection of publications are available in Spanish.

Contact info. phone: 877-NCCS-YES (877-622-7937), **e-mail:** info@canceradvocacy.org, **website:** http://canceradvocacy.org

Appendix

Converting to Metrics

Measurement Conversions

We have included the following tables so you can easily convert measuring ingredients.

Volume Measurement Conversions	
U.S.	**Metric**
¼ teaspoon	1.25 ml
½ teaspoon	2.5 ml
¾ teaspoon	3.75 ml
1 teaspoon	5 ml
1 tablespoon	15 ml
¼ cup	62.5 ml
½ cup	125 ml
¾ cup	187.5 ml
1 cup	250 ml

Weight Conversion Measurements	
U.S.	**Metric**
1 ounce	28.4 g
8 ounces	227.5 g
16 ounces (1 pound)	455 g

Temperature Conversions

We've also included the following table and calculations so you can easily convert cooking temperatures for our recipes.

Cooking Temperature Conversions	
Celsius/Centigrade	0°C and 100°C are arbitrarily placed at the melting and boiling points of water and standard to the metric system
Fahrenheit	Fahrenheit established 0°F as the stabilized temperature when equal amounts of ice, water, and salt are mixed.

To convert temperatures in Fahrenheit to Celsius, use this formula:

$$C = (F - 32) \times 0.5555$$

So, for example, if you are baking at 350°F and want to know that temperature in Celsius, use this calculation:

$$C = (350 - 32) \times 0.5555 = 176.66°C$$

References

Chapter 1: Understanding Cancer and Reducing Your Risk

A Report of the Surgeon General, Physical Activity and Health, U.S. Department of Health and Human Services. Centers for Disease Control and Prevention, National Center for Chronic Disease Prevention and Health Promotion, The President's Council on Physical Fitness and Sports, cdc.gov/nccdphp/sgr/contents.htm.

Ajani, U., M. Gaziano, P. Lotufo, S. Liu, C. Hennekens, and J. Manson. "Alcohol Intake and Risk of Coronary Heart Disease by Diabetes Status." *Circulation* 102 (2000): 500–505.

Alcohol and Cancer. American Cancer Society, February 2002, cancer .org/downloads/pvo/alcohol.pdf.

Calle, E. E., C. Rodriguez, K. Walker-Thurmond, and J. M. Thun. "Overweight, Obesity and Mortality from Cancer in a Prospectively Studied Cohort of U.S. Adults." *New England Journal of Medicine* 348 (2003): 1625–38.

Cannon, L., D. T. Bishop, M. Skolnick, et al. "Genetic Epidemiology of Prostate Cancer in the Utah Mormon Genealogy." *Cancer Survey* 1 (1982): 47–69.

Carter, B. S., T. H. Beaty, G. D. Steinberg, et al. "Mendelian Inheritance of Familial Prostate Cancer. *Proceedings of the National Academy of Sciences of the United States of America* 89 (1992): 3367–71.

Centers for Disease Control and Prevention. "Alcohol-Attributable Deaths and Years of Potential Life Lost—United States, 2001." *Morbidity and Mortality Weekly Report* 53 (Sep. 24, 2004): 866–70.

Chen, W. Y., G. A. Colditz, B. Rosner, S. E. Hankinson, D. J. Hunter, J. E. Manson, M. J. Stampfer, W. C. Willett, and F. E. Speizer. "Use of Postmenopausal Hormones, Alcohol, and Risk for Invasive Breast Cancer." *Annals of Internal Medicine* 137 (Nov. 19, 2002): 798–804.

Dietary Guidelines for Americans. U.S. Department of Agriculture, U.S. Department of Health and Human Services. Accessed Mar. 12, 2003, healthierus.gov/dietaryguidelines.

Dufour, M.C. "What Is Moderate Drinking? Defining 'Drinks' and Drinking Levels." *Alcohol Research and Health: The Journal of the National Institute on Alcohol Abuse and Alcoholism* 23 (1999): 5–14.

Eaton, S. B., and S. B. Eaton III. "Paleolithic vs. Modern Diets— Selected Pathophysiological Implications." *European Journal of Nutrition* 39 (Apr. 2000): 67–70.

Ford, E., D. Williamson, and S. Liu. "Weight Change and Diabetes Incidence: Findings from a National Cohort of U.S. Adults." *American Journal of Epidemiology* (1997): 146.

Fung, T., F. B. Hu, C. Fuchs, E. Giovannucci, D. J. Hunter, M. J. Stampfer, G. A. Colditz, and W. C. Willett. "Major Dietary Patterns and the Risk of Colorectal Cancer in Women." *Archives of Internal Medicine* 163 (2003): 309–14.

Ghadirian, P., G. R. Howe, T. G. Hislop, et al. "Family History of Prostate Cancer: A Multi-Center Case-Control Study in Canada." *International Journal of Cancer* 70 (1997): 679–81.

Giovannucci, E. "Insulin and Colon Cancer." *Cancer Causes Control* 6 (1995): 164–79.

Goldberg, I. J., L. Mosca, M. R. Piano, and E. A. Fisher. "AHA Science Advisory: Wine and Your Heart: A Science Advisory for Healthcare Professionals from the Nutrition Committee, Council on Epidemiology and Prevention, and Council on Cardiovascular Nursing of the American Heart Association." *Circulation* 103 (2001): 472–75.

Grönberg, H., L. Damber, and J. E. Damber. "Familial Prostate Cancer in Sweden. A Nationwide Register Cohort Study." *Cancer* 77 (1996): 138–43.

Hardman, A. E. "Physical Activity and Cancer Risk." *The Proceedings of the Nutrition Society* 60 (Feb. 2001): 107–13.

Harvard Report on Cancer Prevention, Vol. 1: Causes of Human Cancer. *Cancer Causes Control* 7 Supp. (1996): S55–S58.

Harvard Report on Cancer Prevention, Vol. 3: Prevention of Colon Cancer in the United States. *Cancer Causes Control* 10 (1999): 167–80.

He, K., F. B. Hu, G. A. Colditz, J. E. Manson, W. C. Willett, and S. Liu. "Changes in Intake of Fruits and Vegetables in Relation to Risk of Obesity and Weight Gain Among Middle-Aged Women." *International Journal of Obesity and Related Metabolic Disorders* 28, no. 12 (Dec. 2004): 1569–74.

Key, T. J., A. Schatzkin, W. C. Willett, N. E. Allen, E. A. Spencer, and R. C. Travis. "Diet, Nutrition and the Prevention of Cancer. *Public Health Nutrition* 7 (Feb. 2004): 187–200.

Lahmann, P. H., K. Hoffmann, N. Allen, et al. "Body Size and Breast Cancer Risk: Findings from the European Prospective Investigation into Cancer and Nutrition (EPIC)." *International Journal of Cancer* 111 (Sep. 20, 2004): 762–71.

Laufer E. M., T. J. Hartman, D. J. Baer, E. W. Gunter, J. F. Dorgan, W. S. Campbell, B. A. Clevidence, E. D. Brown, D. Albanes, J. T. Judd, and P. R. Taylor. "Effects of Moderate Alcohol Consumption on Folate and Vitamin B(12) Status in Postmenopausal Women." *European Journal of Clinical Nutrition* 58 (Nov. 2004): 1518–24.

Leitzmann, M. F., E. L. Giovannucci, M. J. Stampfer, et al. "Prospective Study of Alcohol Consumption Patterns in Relation to Symptomatic Gallstone Disease in Men." *Alcoholism, Clinical and Experimental Research* 23 (1999): 835–41.

Liu, S., I. Lee, P. Linson, U. Ajani, J. Buring, and C. Hennekens. "A Prospective Study of Physical Activity and Risk of Prostate Cancer in U.S. Physicians." *International Journal of Epidemiology* 29 (2000): 29–35.

Liu, S., M. K. Serdula, D. F. Williamson, A. H. Mokdad, and T. Byers. "A Prospective Study of Alcohol Intake and Change in Body Weight Among U.S. Adults." *American Journal of Epidemiology* 140 (1994): 912–20.

Liu, S., P. Z. Siegel, R. D. Brewer, A. H. Mokdad, D. A. Sleet, and M. Serdula. "Prevalence of Alcohol-Impaired Driving. Results from a National Self-Reported Survey of Health Behaviors." *JAMA* 277 (1997): 122–125.

Ludwig, D. S., J. A. Majzoub, A. Al-Zahrani, G. E. Dallal, I. Blanco, and S. B. Roberts. "High Glycemic Index Foods, Overeating and Obesity." *Pediatrics* 103 (Mar. 1999): E26.

Maciel, M. E., G. D. Castro, and J. A. Castro. "Inhibition of the Rat Breast Cytosolic Bioactivation of Ethanol to Acetaldehyde by Some Plant Polyphenols and Folic Acid." *Nutrition and Cancer* 49 (2004): 94–99.

Matikaine, M. P., E. Pukkala, J. Schleutker, et al. "Relatives of Prostate Cancer Patients Have an Increased Risk of Prostate and Stomach Cancers: A Population-Based, Cancer Registry Study in Finland." *Cancer Causes Control* 12 (2001): 223–30.

McCullough, M. L., and E. Giovannucci. "Diet and Cancer Prevention." *Oncogene* 38 (2004): 6349–64.

Moore, L. L., M. L. Bradlee, M. R. Singer, G. L. Splansky, M. H. Proctor, R. C. Ellison, and B. E. Kreger. "BMI and Waist Circumference as Predictors of Lifetime Colon Cancer Risk in Framingham Study Adults." *International Journal of Obesity and Related Metabolic Disorders* 28 (Apr. 2004): 559–67.

Nasca, P. C., S. Liu, M. S. Baptiste, C. S. Kwon, H. Jacobson, and B. B. Metzger. "Alcohol Consumption and Breast Cancer: Estrogen Receptor Status and Histology." *American Journal of Epidemiology* 140 (1994): 980–88.

Nishikawa, A., Y. Mori, I. S. Lee, T. Tanaka, and M. Hirose. "Cigarette Smoking, Metabolic Activation and Carcinogenesis." *Current Drug Metabolism* 5 (Oct. 2004): 363–73

Platz, E. A., W. C. Willett, G. A. Colditz, et al. "Proportion of Colon Cancer Risk That Might Be Preventable in a Cohort of Middle-Aged U.S. Men." *Cancer Causes Control* 11 (2000): 579–88. (cited in Health Professionals Follow Up Study)

Potential Cause of Prostate Cancer Identified (press release). Harvard School of Public Health, Tuesday, September 30, 1997, hsph.harvard.edu/press/releases/press09301997.

Harvard Center for Cancer Prevention. *Prostate Cancer Fact Sheet.* your diseaserisk.harvard.edu.

Ruf, J. C. "Alcohol, Wine and Platelet Function." *Biological Research* 37 (2004): 209–15.

Sasco, A. J., M. B. Secretan, and K. Straif. "Tobacco Smoking and Cancer: A Brief Review of Recent Epidemiological Evidence." *Lung Cancer* 45 (Suppl. 2) (Aug 2004): S3–S9.

Siiteri, P. K. "Adipose Tissue as a Source of Hormones." *American Journal of Clinical Nutrition* 45 (1987): 277–282.

Slattery, M. L., W. Samowitz, K. Ma, M. Murtaugh, C. Sweeny, T. R. Levin, and S. Neuhassen. "CYP1A1, Cigarette Smoking, and Colon and Rectal Cancer." *American Journal of Epidemiology* 160 (Nov. 1, 2004): 842–52.

Stanford, J. L., and E. A. Ostrander. "Familial Prostate Cancer." *Epidemiologic Review* 23 (2001): 19–23.

Sturm, R. "Increases in Clinically Severe Obesity in the United States, 1986–2000." *Archives of Internal Medicine* 163 (2003): 2146–48.

Vastag, B. "Obesity Is Now on Everyone's Plate." *JAMA* 291 (2004): 1186–88.

Wasserman, L., S. W. Flatt, L. Natarajan, et al. "Correlates of Obesity in Postmenopausal Women with Breast Cancer: Comparison of Genetic, Demographic, Disease-Related, Life History and Dietary Factors." *International Journal of Obesity and Related Metabolic Disorders* 28 (Jan. 2004): 49–56.

Willett, W. C. "Diet and Cancer: One View at the Start of the Millennium." *Cancer Epidemiology, Biomarkers and Prevention* 10 (Jan. 2001): 3–8.

World Cancer Research Fund/American Institute for Cancer Research. *Food, Nutrition and the Prevention of Cancer: A Global Perspective.* Washington, DC: American Institute for Cancer Research, 1997.

Zhang, S., D. J. Hunter, S. E. Hankinson, et al. "A Prospective Study of Folate Intake and the Risk of Breast Cancer." *JAMA* 281 (1999): 1632–37.

Zhang, S. M., W. C. Willett, J. Selhub, D. J. Hunter, E. L. Giovannucci, M. D. Holmes, G. A. Colditz, and S. E. Hankinson. "Plasma Folate, Vitamin B_6, Vitamin B_{12}, Homocysteine, and Risk of Breast Cancer." *Journal of the National Cancer Institute* 95 (Mar. 5, 2003): 373–80.

Chapter 2: Diet and Your Diagnosis

American Cancer Society. *Nutrition for the Person with Cancer: A Guide for Patients and Families.* Atlanta, GA: American Cancer Society, 2000.

Harvie, M. N., I. T. Campbell, A. Baildam, et al. "Energy Balance in Early Breast Cancer Patients Receiving Adjuvant Chemotherapy." *Breast Cancer Research and Treatment* 83 (2004): 201–10.

Langstein, H. N., and J. A. Norton. "Mechanisms of Cancer Cachexia." *Hematology/Oncology Clinics of North America* 5 (1991): 103–23.

National Cancer Institute. Nutrition in Cancer Care, PDQ. cancernet .nci.nih.gov/cancertopics/pdq/supportivecare/nutrition.

Ottery, F. D. "Cancer Cachexia: Prevention, Early Diagnosis, and Management." *Cancer Practice* 2 (Mar.–Apr. 1994): 123–31.

Pierce, J., V. A. Newman, S. W. Flatt, et al. "Telephone Counseling Intervention Increases Intakes of Micronutrient- and Phytochemical-Rich Vegetables, Fruit and Fiber in Breast Cancer Survivors." *Journal of Nutrition* 134 (Feb. 2004): 452–58.

Rock, C. "Dietary Counseling Is Beneficial for the Patient with Cancer." *Journal of Clinical Oncology* 23 (Mar. 1, 2005): 1348–49.

Ross, B. T. "Cancer's Impact on the Nutrition Status of Patients." In: Bloch, A. S. *Nutrition Management of the Cancer Patient.* Rockville, MD: Aspen Publishers, 1990, pp. 11–13.

Shils, M. E. "Nutrition and Diet in Cancer Management." In: Shils, M. E., J. A. Olson, M. Shike, et al., eds. *Modern Nutrition in Health and Disease.* 9th ed. Baltimore, MD: Williams & Wilkins, 1999, pp. 1317–47.

Shils, M. E. "Nutrition Needs of Cancer Patients." In: Bloch, A. S. *Nutrition Management of the Cancer Patient.* Rockville, MD: Aspen Publishers, 1990, pp. 3–10.

Tisdale, M. J. "Cancer Cachexia." *Anticancer Drugs* 4 (1993): 115–25.

Vigano, A., S. Watanabe, and E. Bruera. "Anorexia and Cachexia in Advanced Cancer Patients." *Cancer Surveys* 21(1994): 99–115.

Zeman, F. J. "Nutrition and Cancer." *Clinical Nutrition and Dietetics.* 2nd ed. New York, NY: Macmillan, 1991, pp. 571–98.

Chapter 3: Fats, Carbs, and Cancer

Adom, K. K., and R. H. Liu. "Antioxidant Activity of Grains." *Journal of Agricultural and Food Chemistry* 50 (2002): 6182–87.

Adom, K. K., M. E. Sorrells, and R. H. Liu. "Phytochemicals and Antioxidant Activity of Wheat Varieties." *Journal of Agricultural and Food Chemistry* 51 (2003): 7825–34.

Alpha-Tocopherol, Beta Carotene Cancer Prevention Study Group, The. "The Effect of Vitamin E and Beta-Carotene on the Incidence of Lung Cancer and Other Cancers in Male Smokers." *New England Journal of Medicine* 330 (1994): 1029–35.

Augustin, L. S., C. Galeone, L. Dal Maso, C. Pelucchi, V. Ramazzotti, D. J. Jenkins, M. Montella, R. Talamini, E. Negri, S. Franceschi, and C. La Vecchia. "Glycemic Index, Glycemic Load and Risk of Prostate Cancer." *International Journal of Cancer* 112 (Nov. 10, 2004): 446–50.

Augustin, L. S., S. Gallus, E. Negri, and C. La Vecchia. "Glycemic Index, Glycemic Load and Risk of Gastric Cancer." *Annals of Oncology* 15 (Apr. 2004): 581–84.

Blot, W. J., J. Y. Li, P. R. Taylor, W. Guo, S. Dawsey, G. Q. Wang, C. S. Yang, S. F. Zheng, M. Gail, et al. "Nutrition Intervention Trials in Linxian, China: Supplementation with Specific Vitamin/Mineral Combinations, Cancer Incidence, and Disease-Specific Mortality in the General Population." *Journal of the National Cancer Institute* 85 (1993): 1483–92.

Brand, J. C., P. L. Nicholson, A. W. Thorburn, and A. S. Truswell. "Food Processing and the Glycemic Index." *American Journal of Clinical Nutrition* 42 (1985): 1192–96.

Chatenoud, L., C. La Vecchia, S. Franceschi, A. Tavani, D. R. Jacobs, Jr., M. T. Parpinel, M. Soler, and E. Negri. "Refined-Cereal Intake and Risk of Selected Cancers in Italy." *American Journal of Clinical Nutrition* 70 (Dec. 1999): 1107–10.

Cho, E., D. Spiegelman, D. J. Hunter, W. Y. Chen, G. A. Colditz, and W. C. Willett. "Premenopausal Dietary Carbohydrate, Glycemic Index, Glycemic Load, and Fiber in Relation to Risk of Breast Cancer." *Cancer Epidemiology, Biomarkers and Prevention* 12 (Nov. 2003): 1153–58.

Cho, E., D. Spiegelman, D. J. Hunter, W. Y. Chen, M. J. Stampfer, G. A. Colditz, and W. C. Willett. "Premenopausal Fat Intake and Risk of Breast Cancer." *Journal of the National Cancer Institute* 95 (July 16, 2003): 1079–85.

Chu, Y.-F., J. Sun, X. Wu, and R.H. Liu. "Antioxidant and Antiproliferative Activities of Vegetables." *Journal of Agricultural and Food Chemistry* 50 (2002): 6910–16.

Duncan, A. M. "The Role of Nutrition in the Prevention of Breast Cancer." *AACN Clinical Issues* 15 (Jan.-Mar. 2004): 119–35.

Field, C. J., and P. D. Schley. "Evidence for Potential Mechanisms for the Effect of Conjugated Linoleic Acid on Tumor Metabolism and Immune Function: Lessons from n-3 Fatty Acids." *The American*

Journal of Clinical Nutrition 79, (Suppl. 6) (June 2004): 1190S–1198S.

Ford, E., and S. Liu. "Dietary Glycemic Index and Serum High-Density Lipoprotein Cholesterol Concentration Among United States Adults. *Archives of Internal Medicine* 161 (2001): 572–76.

Frazier, A. L., L. Li, E. Cho, W. C. Willett, and G. A. Colditz. "Adolescent Diet and Risk of Breast Cancer." *Cancer Causes Control* 15 (Feb. 2004): 73–82.

Giovannucci, E., E. B. Rimm, G. Colditz, et al. "A Prospective Study of Dietary Fat and Risk of Prostate Cancer." *Journal of the National Cancer Institute* 85 (1993): 1571–79.

Giovannucci, E., M. J. Stampfer, G. Colditz, et al. "Relationship of Diet to Risk of Colorectal Adenoma in Men." *Journal of the National Cancer Institute* 84 (1992): 91–98.

Greenberg, E. R., J. A. Baron, T. A. Stuckel, M. M. Stevens, and J. S. Mandel. "A Clinical Trial of Beta-Carotene to Prevent Basal Cell and Squamous Cell Cancers of the Skin." *New England Journal of Medicine* 323 (1990): 789–95.

Gross, S., L. Li, E. Ford, and S. Liu. "Increased Consumption of Low-Quality Carbohydrates and the Epidemic of Type 2 Diabetes Mellitus in the United States: An Ecological Assessment." *American Journal of Clinical Nutrition* 79 (2004): 774–79.

Hallfrisch, J., FACN, and K. M. Behall. "Mechanisms of the Effects of Grains on Insulin and Glucose Responses." *Journal of the American College of Nutrition* 19 (2000): 320S–325S.

Hardman, W. E. "(N-3) Fatty Acids and Cancer Therapy." *Journal of Nutrition* 134, (Suppl. 12) (Dec. 2004): 3427S–3430S.

Heller, A. R., T. Rossel, B. Gottschlich, O. Tiebel, M. Menschikowski, R. J. Litz, T. Zimmermann, and T. Koch. "Omega-3 Fatty Acids Improve Liver and Pancreas Function in Postoperative Cancer Patients." *International Journal of Cancer* 111, no. 4 (Sept. 10, 2004): 611–16.

Hennekens, C. H., J. E. Buring, J. E. Manson, M. Stampfer, and B. Rosner. "Lack of Effect of Long-Term Supplementation with Beta-

Carotene on the Incidence of Malignant Neoplasms and Cardiovascular Disease." *New England Journal of Medicine* 334 (1996): 1145–49.

Higginbotham, S., Z. Zhang, I. Lee, N. Cook, J. Buring, and S. Liu. "Dietary Glycemic Load and Breast Cancer Risk in the Women's Health Study." *Cancer Epidemiology, Biomarkers and Prevention* 13 (2004): 65–70.

Higginbotham, S., Z. Zhang, I. Lee, N. Cook, E. Giovannucci, J. Buring, S. Liu. "Dietary Glycemic Load and Colon Cancer Risk in the Women's Health Study." *Journal of the National Cancer Institute* 96 (2004): 121–29.

Holmes, M., S. Liu, S. Hankinson, D. Hunter, and W. Willett. "Dietary Fiber, Carbohydrates and Breast Cancer Risk." *American Journal of Epidemiology* 159 (2004): 732–39.

Howe, G. R., K. J. Aronson, E. Benito, et al. "The Relationship Between Dietary Fat Intake and Risk of Colorectal Cancer-Evidence from the Combined Analysis of 13 Case-Control Studies." *Cancer Causes Control* 8 (1997): 215–28.

Howe, G. R., T. Hirohata, T. G. Hislop, J. M. Iscovich, J. M. Yuan, K. Katsouyanni, et al. "Dietary Factors and Risk of Breast Cancer: Combined Analysis of 12 Case-Control Studies." *Journal of the National Cancer Institute* 82 (1990): 561–69.

Hu, F. B., J. E. Manson, S. Liu, D. Hunter, G. A. Colditz, K. B. Michels, F. E. Speizer, and E. Giovannucci. "Prospective Study of Adult Onset Diabetes Mellitus (Type 2) and Risk of Colorectal Cancer in Women." *Journal of the National Cancer Institute* 91 (1999): 542.

Institute of Medicine. *Dietary Reference for Intakes for Energy, Carbohydrate, Fiber, Fat, Fatty Acids, Cholesterol, Protein, and Amino Acids.* Washington, DC: National Academies Press, 2002.

Jenkins, D. J., C. W. Kendall, L. S. Augustin, et al. "Glycemic Index: Overview of Implications in Health and Disease." *American Journal of Clinical Nutrition* 76 (2002): 266S–273S.

Khor, G. L. "Dietary Fat Quality: A Nutritional Epidemiologist's View." *Asia Pacific Journal of Clinical Nutrition* 13 (Suppl.) (Aug. 2004): S22.

Koh-Banerjee, P., M. Franz, L. Sampson, S. Liu, D. Spiegelman, W. Willett, and E. Rimm. "Changes in Whole Grain, Bran, and Cereal Fiber Consumption with 8-Year Weight Gain Among U.S. Male Health Professionals Using New Quantitative Estimates of Whole Grain Intakes." *American Journal of Clinical Nutrition* 80 (2004): 1237–24.

Kushi, L., and E. Giovannucci. "Dietary Fat and Cancer." *American Journal of Medicine* 113 (Suppl. 9B) (2002): 63S–70S.

Larsson, S. C., M. Kumlin, M. Ingelman-Sundberg, and A. Wolk. "Dietary Long Chain Omega-3 Fatty Acids for the Prevention of Cancer: A Review of Potential Mechanisms." *American Journal of Clinical Nutrition* 79 (June 2004): 935–45.

Lásztity, R. *Cereal Chemistry.* Budapest: Akadémiai Kiadó, 1999.

Levi, F., C. Pasche, F. Lucchini, L. Chatenoud, D. R. Jacobs, Jr., and C. La Vecchia. "Refined and Whole Grain Cereals and the Risk of Oral, Oesophageal and Laryngeal Cancer." *European Journal of Clinical Nutrition* 54 (June 2000): 487–89.

Levi, F., C. Pasche, F. Lucchini, and C. LaVecchia. "Macronutrients and Colorectal Cancer: A Swiss Case-Control Study." *Annals of Oncology: Official Journal of the European Society for Medical Oncology/ESMO* 13, no. 3 (March 2002): 369–73.

Liu, S. "Insulin Resistance, Hyperglycemia and Risk of Major Chronic Diseases—A Dietary Perspective." *Procedings of the Nutrition Society of Australia* 22 (1998): 140–50.

Liu, S. "Intake of Refined Carbohydrates and Whole Grain Foods in Relation to Risk of Type 2 Diabetes Mellitus and Coronary Heart Disease." *Journal of the American College of Nutrition* 21 (2002): 298–306.

Liu, S., J. Buring, H. Sesso, E. Rimm, W. C. Willett, and J. Manson. "A Prospective Study of Dietary Fiber Intake and Risk of Cardiovascular Disease Among Women." *Journal of the American College of Cardiology* 39 (2002): 49–56.

Liu, S., I. Lee, U. Ajani, S. Cole, J. Buring, and J. Manson. "Intake of Vegetables Rich in Carotenoids and Risk of Coronary Heart Disease in Men: The Physicians' Health Study." *International Journal of Epidemiology* 30 (2001): 130–35.

Liu, S., J. Manson, J. Buring, M. Stampfer, W. C. Willett, and P. Ridker. "Relation Between a Diet with a High Glycemic Load and Plasma Concentrations of High-Sensitivity C-Reactive Protein in Middle-Aged Women." *American Journal of Clinical Nutrition* 75 (2002): 492–98.

Liu, S., J. Manson, I. Lee, S. Cole, W. C. Willett, and J. Buring. "Fruit and Vegetable Intake and Risk of Cardiovascular Disease: The Women's Health Study." *American Journal of Clinical Nutrition* 72 (2000): 922–28.

Liu, S., J. E. Manson, M. Stampfer, M. D. Holmes, F. B. Hu, S. E. Hankinson, and W. C. Willett. "Dietary Glycemic Load Assessed by Food Frequency Questionnaire in Relation to Plasma High-Density Lipoprotein Cholesterol and Fasting Triglycerides Among Postmenopausal Women." *American Journal of Clinical Nutrition* 73 (2001): 560–66.

Liu, S., J. E. Manson, M. J. Stampfer, F. B. Hu, E. Giovannucci, G. A. Colditz, C. H. Hennekens, and W. C. Willett. "A Prospective Study of Whole-Grain Intake and Risk of Type 2 Diabetes Mellitus in U.S. Women." *American Journal of Public Health* 90 (2000): 1409–15.

Liu, S., J. E. Manson, M. J. Stampfer, K. M. Rexrode, F. B. Hu, E. B. Rimm, and W. C. Willett. "Whole Grain Consumption and Risk of Ischemic Stroke in Women: A Prospective Study." *JAMA* 284 (2000):1534–40.

Liu, S., H. Sesso, J. Manson, W. C. Willett, and J. Buring. "Is Intake of Breakfast Cereal Related to Total and Cause-Specific Mortality in Men?" *American Journal of Clinical Nutrition* 77 (2003): 595–99.

Liu, S., M. Stampfer, F. Hu, E. Giovannucci, E. Rimm, J. Manson, C. Hennekens, and W. C. Willett. "Whole Grain Consumption and

Risk of Coronary Heart Disease: Results from the Nurses' Health Study." *American Journal of Clinical Nutrition* 70 (1999): 412–19.

Liu, S., W. C. Willett, J. Manson, F. Hu, B. Rosner, and G. Colditz. "Changes in Intake of Dietary Fiber and Grain Products in Relation to Changes in Weight and the Development of Obesity Among Middle-Aged Women." *American Journal of Clinical Nutrition* 78 (2003): 920–27.

Liu, S., W. C. Willett, M. J. Stampfer, et al. "A Prospective Study of Dietary Glycemic Load, Carbohydrate Intake and Risk of Coronary Heart Disease in U.S. Women." *American Journal of Clinical Nutrition* 71 (2000): 1455–61.

Lu, Q. Y., J. R. Arteaga, Q. Zhang, S. Huerta, V. L. Go, and D. Heber. "Inhibition of Prostate Cancer Cell Growth by an Avocado Extract: Role of Lipid-Soluble Bioactive Substances." *The Journal of Nutritional Biochemistry* 16, no. 1 (Jan. 2005): 23–30.

Ludwig, D. "Dietary Glycemic Index and Obesity." *Journal of Nutrition* 130 (2000): 280S–283S.

Martin-Moreno, J. M., W. C. Willett, L. Gorgojo, et al. "Dietary Fat, Olive Oil Intake and Breast Cancer Risk." *International Journal of Cancer* 58 (1994): 774–80.

McKeown, N., J. Meigs, S. Liu, E. Saltzman, P. Wilson, and P. Jacques. "Carbohydrate Nutrition, Insulin Resistance, and the Prevalence of the Insulin Resistance Syndrome in the Framingham Offspring Cohort." *Diabetes Care* 27 (2004): 538–546.

McKeown, N. M., J. B. Meigs, S. Liu, P. W. Wilson, and P. F. Jacques. "Whole-Grain Intake Is Favorably Associated with Metabolic Risk Factors for Type 2 Diabetes and Cardiovascular Disease in the Framingham Offspring Study." *American Journal of Clinical Nutrition* 76 (2002): 390–98.

Michaud, D., S. Liu, E. Giovannucci, W. C. Willett, G. Colditz, and C. Fuchs. "Dietary Glycemic Load, Carbohydrate, Sucrose and Risk of Pancreatic Cancer in a Prospective Study of Women." *Journal of the National Cancer Institute* 94 (2002): 1293–1300.

National Institutes of Health. *NIH Consensus Development Conference Statement on Diet and Exercise.* Bethesda, MD: U.S. Department of Health and Human Services, 1986.

Oh, K., W. C. Willett, C. S. Fuchs, and E. L. Giovannucci. "Glycemic Index, Glycemic Load, and Carbohydrate Intake in Relation to Risk of Distal Colorectal Adenoma in Women." *Cancer Epidemiology, Biomarkers and Prevention* 13 (Jul. 2004): 1192–98.

Omenn, G. S., G. E. Goodman, M. D. Thomquist, J. Barnes, and M. R. Cullen. "Effects of a Combination of Beta-Carotene and Vitamin A on Lung Cancer and Cardiovascular Disease." *New England Journal of Medicine* 334 (1996): 1150–55.

Outwater, J. L., A. Nicholson, and N. Barnard. "Dairy Products and Breast Cancer: The IGF-1, Estrogen, and bGH Hypothesis." *Medical Hypotheses* 48 (1997): 453–61.

Potential Cause of Prostate Cancer Identified (press release). Harvard School of Public Health, Tues. Sept. 30, 1997, hsph.harvard.edu/press/releases/press09301997.

Roynette, C. E., P. C. Calder, Y. M. Dupertuis, and C. Pichard. "N-3 Polyunsaturated Fatty Acids and Colon Cancer Prevention." *Clinical Nutrition* 23, no. 2 (April 2004): 139–51.

Salonen, J. T., K. Nyyssonen, R. Salonen, H. M. Lakka, J. Kaikkonen, E. Porkkala-Sarataho, S. Voutilainen, T. A. Lakka, T. Rissanen, et al. "Antioxidant Supplementation in Artherosclerosis Prevention (ASAP) Study: A Randomized Trial of the Effect of Vitamins E and C on 3-Year Progression of Carotid Atherosclerosis." *Journal of Internal Medicine* 248 (2000): 377–86.

Schley, P. D., H. B. Jijon, L. E. Robinson, and C. J. Field. "Mechanisms of Omega-3 Fatty Acid–Induced Growth Inhibition in MDA-MB-231 Human Breast Cancer Cells." *Breast Cancer Research and Treatment* 92, no. 2 (July 2005): 187–95.

Sieri, S., V. Krogh, V. Pala, et al. "Dietary Patterns and Risk of Breast Cancer in the ORDET Cohort." *Cancer Epidemiology, Biomarkers and Prevention* 13 (2004): 567–72.

Simopoulos, A. P. "The Traditional Diet of Greece and Cancer." *European Journal of Cancer* 13 (June 2004): 219–30.

Slattery, M., J. Benson, K. N. Ma, D. Shafer, and J. D. Potter. "Trans Fatty Acids and Colon Cancer." *Nutrition and Cancer* 39 (2001): 170–75.

Slavin, J. L. "Mechanisms for the Impact of Whole Grain Foods on Cancer Risk." *Journal of the American College of Nutrition* 19 (June 2000): 300S–307S.

Stephens, N. G., A. Parsons, P. M. Schofield, F. Kelly, K. Cheeseman, and M. J. Mitchinson. "Randomized Controlled Trial of Vitamin E in Patients with Coronary Disease: Cambridge Heart Antioxidant Study (CHAOS)." *Lancet* 347 (1996): 781–86.

Sukocheva, O. A., Y. Yang, J. F. Gierthy, and R. F. Seegal. "Methyl Mercury Influences Growth-Related Signaling in MCF-7 Breast Cancer Cells." *Environmental Toxicology* 20, no. 1 (Feb. 2005): 32–44.

Sun, J., Y. F. Chu, X. Wu, and R. H. Liu. "Antioxidant and Antiproliferative Activities of Fruits." *Journal of Agricultural and Food Chemistry* 50 (2002): 7449–54.

Terry, P. D., M. Jain, A. B. Miller, G. R. Howe, and T. E. Rohan. "Glycemic Load, Carbohydrate Intake, and Risk of Colorectal Cancer in Women: A Prospective Cohort Study." *Journal of the National Cancer Institute* 95 (2003): 914–16.

Trichopoulou, A., K. Katsouyanni, S. Stuver, et al. "Consumption of Olive Oil and Specific Food Groups in Relation to Breast Cancer Risk in Greece." *Journal of the National Cancer Institute* 87 (1995): 110–16.

"What You Need to Know About Mercury in Fish and Shellfish." 2004 EPA and FDA advice, cfsan.fda.gov/~dms/admehg3.

Willett, W. C. "Goals for Nutrition in the Year 2000." *CA: A Cancer Journal* 49 (Nov.–Dec. 1999): 331–52.

Willett, W. C., M. J. Stampfer, G. A. Colditz, et al. "Relation of Meat, Fat and Fiber Intake to the Risk of Colon Cancer in a Prospective Study Among Women." *New England Journal of Medicine* 323 (1990): 1664–72.

Wolever, T., and C. Bolognesi. "Prediction of Glucose and Insulin Responses of Normal Subjects After Consuming Mixed Meals Varying in Energy, Protein, Fat, Carbohydrate and Glycemic Index." *Nutrition* 126 (1992): 2807–12.

Wolever, T. M., D. J. Jenkins, A. L. Jenkins, and R. G. Josse. "The Glycemic Index: Methodology and Clinical Implications." *American Journal of Clinical Nutrition* 54 (1991): 846–54.

World Cancer Research Fund, American Institute for Cancer Research. "Food, Nutrition and the Prevention of Cancer: A Global Perspective." *Breast*. Washington, DC: American Institute for Cancer Research, 1997, pp. 252–87.

Wynter, M. P., S. T. Russell, and J. J. Tisdale. "Effect of n-3 Fatty Acids on the Antitumour Effects of Cytotoxic Drugs." *In Vivo* 18, no. 5 (Sept.–Oct. 2004): 543–47.

Yusuf, S., G. Dagenais, J. Pogue, J. Bosch, and P. Sleight. "Vitamin E Supplementation and Cardiovascular Events in High-Risk Patients. The Heart Outcomes Prevention Evaluation Study Investigators." *New England Journal of Medicine* 342 (2000): 154–60.

Chapter 4: Antioxidants, Phytonurients, and Other Cancer-Fighting Nutrients

Adom, K. K., and R. H. Liu. "Antioxidant Activity of Grains." *Journal of Agricultural and Food Chemistry* 50 (2002): 6182–87.

Adom, K. K., M. E. Sorrells, and R. H. Liu. "Phytochemicals and Antioxidant Activity of Wheat Varieties." *Journal of Agricultural and Food Chemistry* 51 (2003): 7825–34.

Alpha-Tocopherol, Beta Carotene Cancer Prevention Study Group, The. "The Effect of Vitamin E and Beta-Carotene on the Incidence of Lung Cancer and Other Cancers in Male Smokers." *New England Journal of Medicine* 330 (1994): 1029–35.

Ames, B. N., and L. S. Gold. "Endogenous Mutagens and the Causes of Aging and Cancer." *Mutation Research* 250 (1991): 3–16.

Awad, A. B., and C. S. Fink. "Phytosterols as Anticancer Dietary Components: Evidence and Mechanism of Action." *Journal of Nutrition* 130 (Sep. 2000): 2127–30.

Beatty, S., H. Koh, M. Phil, D. Henson, and M. Boulton. "The Role of Oxidative Stress in the Pathogenesis of Age-Related Macular Degeneration." *Survey of Ophthalmology* 45 (Sep.-Oct. 2000): 115–34.

Benbrook, C. Elevating Antioxidant Levels in Food Through Organic Farming and Food Processing. An Organic State of Science Review. January 2005, organic-center.org/science.htm?article=54.

Berr, C., B. Balansard, J. Arnaud, A. M. Roussel, and A. Alperovitch. "Cognitive Decline Is Associated with Systemic Oxidative Stress: The EVA Study." *Journal of the American Geriatric Society* 48 (Oct. 2000): 1285–91.

Blot, W. J., J. Y. Li, P. R. Taylor, W. Guo, S. Dawsey, G. Q. Wang, C. S. Yang, S. F. Zheng, M. Gail, et al. "Nutrition Intervention Trials in Linxian, China: Supplementation with Specific Vitamin/Mineral Combinations, Cancer Incidence, and Disease-Specific Mortality in the General Population." *Journal of the National Cancer Institute* 85 (1993): 1483–92.

Chen, J., P. M. Stavro, and L. U. Thompson. "Dietary Flaxseed Inhibits Human Breast Cancer Growth and Metastasis and Downregulates Expression of Insulin-Like Growth Factor and Epidural Growth Factor Receptor." *Nutrition and Cancer* 43, no. 2 (2002): 187–92.

Chen, J., E. Hui, T. Ip, and L. U. Thompson. "Dietary Flaxseed Enhances the Inhibitory Effect of Tamoxifen on the Growth of Estrogen-Dependent Human Breast Cancer (MCF-7) in Nude Mice." *Clinical Cancer Research: An Official Journal of the American Association for Cancer Research* 10, vol 22 (Nov. 15, 2004): 7703–11.

Chu, Y.-F., J. Sun, X. Wu, and R. H. Liu. "Antioxidant and Antiproliferative Activities of Vegetables." *Journal of Agricultural and Food Chemistry* 50 (2002): 6910–16.

Dabrosin, C., J. Chen, L. Wang, and L. U. Thompson. "Flaxseed Inhibits Metastasis and Decreases Extracellular Vascular Endothelial

Growth Factor in Human Breast Cancer Xenografts." *Cancer Letters* 185, no. 1 (Nov. 2002): 31–37.

Drewnowski, A., and C. Gomez-Carneros. "Bitter Taste, Phytonutrients, and the Consumer: A Review." *American Journal of Clinical Nutrition* 72 (Dec. 2000): 1424–35.

Eberhardt, M. V., C. Y. Lee, and R. H. Liu. "Antioxidant Activity of Fresh Apples." *Nature* 405 (2000): 903–4.

Elson, C. E. "Suppression of Mevalonate Pathway Activities by Dietary Isoprenoids: Protective Roles in Cancer and Cardiovascular Disease." *Journal of Nutrition* 125 (1995): 1666S–1672S.

Ford, E., S. Liu, D. Mannino, W. Giles, and S. Smith. "C-Reactive Protein Concentration and Concentrations of Blood Vitamins, Carotenoids, and Selenium Among United States Adults." *European Journal of Clinical Nutrition* 57 (2003): 1157–63.

Ford, E., A. Mokdad, U. Ajani, and S. Liu. "Associations Between Concentrations of Alpha- and Gamma-Tocopherol and Concentrations of Glucose, Glycosylated Hemoglobin, Insulin, and C-Peptide Among U.S. Adults." *British Journal of Nutrition* 92 (2004): 1–8.

Greenberg, E. R., J. A. Baron, T. A. Stuckel, M. M. Stevens, and J. S. Mandel. "A Clinical Trial of Beta-Carotene to Prevent Basal Cell and Squamous Cell Cancers of the Skin." *New England Journal of Medicine* 323 (1990): 789–95.

Guthrie, N. and K. K. Carroll. "Inhibition of Mammary Cancer by Citrus Flavonoids." *Advances in Experimental Medicine and Biology* 439 (1998): 227–36.

Harvard School of Public Health, Division of Cancer Prevention. "Taking Antioxidants for Cancer Prevention: A Leap of Faith," hsph.harvard.edu/cancer/publications/source/v9n1/focus

Heber, D., and S. Bowerman. "Applying Science to Changing Dietary Patterns." *Journal of Nutrition* 131 (Nov. 2001): 3078S–3081S.

Heber, D., and S. Bowerman. "Applying Science to Changing Dietary Patterns." *The Journal of Nutrition* 131, (Suppl. 11) (Nov. 2001): 3078S–3081S.

Hennekens, C. H., J. E. Buring, J. E. Manson, M. Stampfer, and B. Rosner. "Lack of Effect of Long-Term Supplementation with Beta-Carotene on the Incidence of Malignant Neoplasms and Cardiovascular Disease." *New England Journal of Medicine* 334 (1996): 1145–49.

Hou, D. X., M. Fujii, N. Terahara, and M. Yoshimoto. "Molecular Mechanisms Behind the Chemopreventive Effects of Anthocyanidins." *Journal of Biomedicine and Biotechnology* 5 (2004): 321–25.

Lee, I. M., N. R. Cook, J. E. Manson. "Beta-Carotene Supplementation and Incidence of Cancer and Cardiovascular Disease: Women's Health Study." *Journal of the National Cancer Institute* 91 (1999) 2102–6.

Liu, R. H. "Health Benefits of Fruits and Vegetables Are from Additive and Synergistic Combination of Phytochemicals." *American Journal of Clinical Nutrition* 78 (2003): 517S–520S.

Liu, R. "Potential Synergy of Phytochemicals in Cancer Prevention: Mechanism of Action." *Journal of Nutrition* 134 (Dec. 2004): 3479S–3485S.

Murillo, G., and R. G. Mehta. "Cruciferous Vegetables and Cancer Prevention." *Nutrition and Cancer* 41 (2001): 17–28.

Nakatani, N. "Chemistry of Antioxidants from *Labiatae* Herbs." In: Huang, M. T., T. Osawa, C. T. Ho, and R. T. Rosen, eds. *Food Phytochemicals for Cancer Prevention II. Teas, Spices and Herbs.* Washington, DC: American Chemical Society, 1994, pp. 144–53.

National Cancer Institute. Antioxidants and Cancer Prevention: Questions and Answers. nci.gov.

National Cancer Institute. "5-A-Day: Glossary of Phytochemicals." 5aday.com/html/consumers/healthcolors.php.

National Institute on Aging. Age Page: Life Extension: Science or Science Fiction? U.S. Department of Health and Human Services, Public Health Service, National Institutes of Health. nih.gov.

National Institute on Aging. Research Goal B: Understand Healthy Aging Processes Subgoal 1: Unlock The Secrets of Aging, Health, and Longevity. nih.gov.

Omenn, G. S., G. Goodman, M. Thomquist, et al. "The Beta-Carotene and Retinol Efficacy Trial (CARET) for Chemoprevention of Lung Cancer in High Risk Populations: Smokers and Asbestos-Exposed Workers." *Cancer Research* 54 (1994): 2038s–2043s.

Omenn, G. S., G. E. Goodman, M. D. Thomquist, J. Barnes, and M. R. Cullen. "Effects of a Combination of Beta-Carotene and Vitamin A on Lung Cancer and Cardiovascular Disease." *New England Journal of Medicine* 334 (1996): 1150–55.

Qureshi, A. A., H. Mo, L. Packer, and D. M. Peterson. "Isolation and Identification of Novel Tocotrienols from Rice Bran with Hypocholesterolemic, Antioxidant, and Antitumor Properties." *Journal of Agricultural and Food Chemistry* 48 (Aug. 2000): 3130–40.

Salonen, J. T., K. Nyyssonen, R. Salonen, H. M. Lakka, J. Kaikkonen, E. Porkkala-Sarataho, S. Voutilainen, T. A. Lakka, T. Rissanen, et al. "Antioxidant Supplementation in Artherosclerosis Prevention (ASAP) Study: A Randomized Trial of the Effect of Vitamins E and C on 3-Year Progression of Carotid Atherosclerosis." *Journal of Internal Medicine* 248 (2000): 377–86.

Sang, S., H. Kikuzaki, K. Lapsley, R. T. Rosen, N. Nakatani, and C. T. Ho. "Sphingolipid and Other Constituents from Almond Nuts (*Prunus amygdalus Batsch*). *Journal of Agricultural and Food Chemistry* 50 (July 31, 2002): 4709–12.

Soliman, K. F., and E. A. Mazzio. "In Vitro Attenuation of Nitric Oxide Production in C6 Astrocyte Cell Culture by Various Dietary Compounds." *Proceedings of the Society for Experimental Biology and Medicine* 218 (Sep. 1998): 390–97.

Steinmetz, K. A., and J. D. Potter. "Vegetables, Fruit and Cancer Prevention: A Review. *Journal of the American Dietetic Association* 96 (Oct. 1996): 1027–39.

Stephens, N. G., A. Parsons, P. M. Schofield, F. Kelly, K. Cheeseman, and M. J. Mitchinson. "Randomized Controlled Trial of Vitamin E in Patients with Coronary Disease: Cambridge Heart Antioxidant Study (CHAOS)." *Lancet* 347 (1996): 781–86.

Sun, J., Y. F. Chu, X. Wu, and R. H. Liu. "Antioxidant and Antiproliferative Activities of Fruits." *Journal of Agricultural and Food Chemistry* 50 (2002): 7449–54.

Temple, N. J., and K. K. Gladwin. "Fruits, Vegetables, and the Prevention of Cancer: Research Challenges." *Nutrition* 19 (2003): 467–70.

U.S. Department of Agriculture, Agricultural Research Service. *Food and Nutrient Intakes by Individuals in the United States, by Sex and Age, 1994–1996.* Nationwide Food Surveys Report No. 96-2. Washington, DC: USDA, 1998.

Verhoeven, D. T. H., R. A. Goldbohm, G. van Poppel, H. Verhagen, and P. A. van den Brandt. "Epidemiological Studies on Brassica Vegetables and Cancer Risk." *Cancer Epidemiology, Biomarkers and Prevention* 5 (1996): 733–48.

Waters, M. D., H. F. Stack, M. A. Jackson, H. E. Brockman, and S. De Flora. "Activity Profiles of Antimutagens: In Vitro and In Vivo Data." *Mutation Research* 19 (Feb. 1996): 109–29.

World Cancer Research Fund/American Institute for Cancer Research. *Food, Nutrition and the Prevention of Cancer: A Global Perspective.* Washington, DC: American Institute for Cancer Research, 1997.

Wu, X., G. R. Beecher, J. M. Holden, D. B. Haytowitz, S. E. Gephardt, and R. L. Prior. "Lipophilic and Hydrophilic Antioxidant Capacities of Common Foods in the United States." *Journal of Agricultural and Food Chemistry* 52 (June 9, 2004): 4026–37.

Yusuf, S., G. Dagenais, J. Pogue, J. Bosch, and P. Sleight. "Vitamin E Supplementation and Cardiovascular Events in High-Risk Patients. The Heart Outcomes Prevention Evaluation Study Investigators." *New England Journal of Medicine* 342 (2000): 154–60.

Zhang, S., X. Yang, and M. E. Morris. "Combined Effects of Multiple Flavonoids on Breast Cancer Resistance Protein (ABCG2)-Mediated Transport." *Pharmaceutical Research* 21, no. 7 (July 2004): 1263–73.

Chapter 5: Cancer-Fighting Foods

Adom, K. K., and R. H. Liu. "Antioxidant Activity of Grains." *Journal of Agricultural and Food Chemistry* 50 (2002): 6182–87.

Adom, K. K., M. E. Sorrells, and R. H. Liu. "Phytochemicals and Antioxidant Activity of Wheat Varieties." *Journal of Agricultural and Food Chemistry* 51 (2003): 7825–34.

Blot, W. J., J. Y. Li, P. R. Taylor, W. Guo, S. Dawsey, G. Q. Wang, C. S. Yang, S. F. Zheng, M. Gail, et. al. "Nutrition Intervention Trials in Linxian, China: Supplementation with Specific Vitamin/Mineral Combinations, Cancer Incidence, and Disease-Specific Mortality in the General Population." *Journal of the National Cancer Institute* 85 (1993): 1483–92.

Chu, Y.-F., J. Sun, X. Wu, and R. H. Liu. "Antioxidant and Antiproliferative Activities of Vegetables." *Journal of Agricultural and Food Chemistry* 50 (2002): 6910–16.

Eberhardt, M. V., C. Y. Lee, and R. H. Liu. "Antioxidant Activity of Fresh Apples." *Nature* 405 (2000): 903–4.

Greenberg, E. R., J. A. Baron, T. A. Stuckel, M. M. Stevens, and J. S. Mandel. "A Clinical Trial of Beta-Carotene to Prevent Basal Cell and Squamous Cell Cancers of the Skin." *New England Journal of Medicine* 323 (1990): 789–95.

Heber, D. "Vegetables, Fruits and Phytoestrogens in the Prevention of Diseases." *Journal of Postgraduate Medicine* 50 (2004): 145–49.

Hennekens, C. H., J. E. Buring, J. E. Manson, M. Stampfer, and B. Rosner. "Lack of Effect of Long-Term Supplementation with Beta-Carotene on the Incidence of Malignant Neoplasms and Cardiovascular Disease." *New England Journal of Medicine* 334 (1996): 1145–49.

Omenn, G. S., G. E. Goodman, M. D. Thomquist, J. Barnes, and M. R. Cullen. "Effects of a Combination of Beta-Carotene and Vitamin A on Lung Cancer and Cardiovascular Disease." *New England Journal of Medicine* 334 (1996): 1150–55.

Salonen, J. T., K. Nyyssonen, R. Salonen, H. M. Lakka, J. Kaikkonen, E. Porkkala-Sarataho, S. Voutilainen, T. A. Lakka, T. Rissanen, et al. "Antioxidant Supplementation in Artherosclerosis Prevention (ASAP) Study: A Randomized Trial of the Effect of Vitamins E and C on 3-Year Progression of Carotid Atherosclerosis." *Journal of Internal Medicine* 248 (2000): 377–86.

Stephens, N. G., A. Parsons, P. M. Schofield, F. Kelly, K. Cheeseman, and M. J. Mitchinson. "Randomized Controlled Trial of Vitamin E in Patients with Coronary Disease: Cambridge Heart Antioxidant Study (CHAOS)." *Lancet* 347 (1996): 781–86.

Sun, J., Y. F. Chu, X. Wu, and R .H. Liu. "Antioxidant and Antiproliferative Activities of Fruits." *Journal of Agricultural and Food Chemistry* 50 (2002): 7449–54.

Yusuf, S., G. Dagenais, J. Pogue, J. Bosch, and P. Sleight. "Vitamin E Supplementation and Cardiovascular Events in High-Risk Patients. The Heart Outcomes Prevention Evaluation Study Investigators." *New England Journal of Medicine* 342 (2000): 154–60.

Chapter 6: Healing Herbs and Spices

Adams, B. K., J. Cai, J. Armstrong, M. Herold, Y. J. Lu, A. Sun, J. P. Snyder, D. C. Liotta, D. P. Jones, and M. Shoji. "EF24, a Novel Synthetic Curcumin Analog, Induces Apoptosis in Cancer Cells via a Redox-Dependent Mechanism." *Anticancer Drugs* 16 (Mar. 2005): 263–75.

Burke, Y. D., M. J. Stark, S. L. Roach, S. E. Sen, and P. L. Crowell. "Inhibition of Pancreatic Cancer Growth by the Dietary Isoprenoids Farnesol and Geraniol." *Lipids* 32 (1997): 151–55.

Choudhuri, T., S. Pal, T. Das, and G. Sa. "Curcumin Selectively Induces Apoptosis in Deregulated Cyclin D1 Expressed Cells at G2 Phase of Cell Cycle in a p53-Dependent Manner." *Journal of Biological Chemistry* 280, no. 20 (May 20, 2005): 20059–68.

Elson, C. E., and S. G. Yu. "The Chemoprevention of Cancer by Mevalonate-Derived Constituents of Fruits and Vegetables." *Journal of Nutrition* 124 (1994): 607–14.

Elson, C. E. "Suppression of Mevalonate Pathway Activities by Dietary Isoprenoids: Protective Roles in Cancer and Cardiovascular Disease." *Journal of Nutrition* 125 (1995): 1666S–1672S.

Furness, M. S., T. P. Robinson, T. Ehlers, R. B. Hubbard IV, J. L. Arbiser, D. J. Goldsmith, and J. P. Bowen. "Antiangiogenic Agents: Studies on Fumagillin and Curcumin Analogs." *Current Pharmaceutical Design* 11 (2005): 357–73.

Katiyar, S. K., N. Ahmad, and H. Mukhtar. "Green Tea and Skin." *Archives of Dermatology* 136 (Aug. 2000): 989–94.

Katiyar, S. K., A. Perez, and H. Mukhtar. "Green Tea Polyphenol Treatment to Human Skin Prevents Formation of Ultraviolet Light B-Induced Pyrimidine Dimers in DNA." *Clinical Cancer Research* 6 (Oct. 2000): 3864–69.

Mukhtar, H., and N. Ahmad. "Tea Polyphenols: Prevention of Cancer and Optimizing Health." *American Journal of Clinical Nutrition* 71 (June 2000): 1698S–1702S.

Nakachi, K., K. Suemasu, K. Suga, T. Takeo, K. Imai, and Y. Higashi. "Influence of Drinking Green Tea on Breast Cancer Malignancy Among Japanese Patients." *Japanese Journal of Cancer Research* 89 (1998): 254–61.

Nakatani, N. "Chemistry of Antioxidants from *Labiatae* Herbs." In: Huang, M. T., T. Osawa, C. T. Ho, and R. T. Rosen, eds. *Food Phytochemicals for Cancer Prevention II. Teas, Spices and Herbs.* Washington, DC: American Chemical Society, 1994, pp. 144–53.

Narayan, S. "Curcumin, a Multi-Functional Chemopreventive Agent, Blocks Growth of Colon Cancer Cells by Targeting Beta-Catenin-Mediated Transactivation and Cell-Cell Adhesion Pathways." *Journal of Molecular Histology* 35 (Mar. 2004): 301–7.

Pearce, B. C., R. A. Parker, M. E. Deason, A. A. Qureshi, and J. J. Wright. "Hypocholesterolemic Activity of Synthetic and Natural

Tocotrienols." *Journal of Medicinal Chemistry* 35 (1992): 3595–3606.

Qureshi, A. A., W. R. Mangels, Z. Z. Din, and C. E. Elson. "Inhibition of Hepatic Mevalonate Biosynthesis by the Monoterpene, d-Limonene." *Journal of Agricultural and Food Chemistry* 36 (1988): 1220–24.

Shenouda, N. S., C. Zhou, J. D. Browning, P. J. Ansell, M. S. Sakla, D. B. Lubahn, and R. S. Macdonald. "Phytoestrogens in Common Herbs Regulate Prostate Cancer Cell Growth in Vitro." *Nutrition and Cancer* 49 (2004): 200–208.

Yu, S. G., N. M. Abuirmeilah, A. A. Qureshi, and C. E. Elson. "Dietary Beta-Ionone Suppresses Hepatic 3-Hydroxy-3-methylglutaryl Coenzyme A Reductase Activity." *Journal of Agricultural and Food Chemistry* 42 (1994): 1493–96.

Yu, S. G., P. J. Anderson, and C. E. Elson. "Efficacy of Beta-Ionone in the Chemoprevention of Rat Mammary Carcinogenesis." *Journal of Agricultural and Food Chemistry* 43 (1995): 2144–47.

Index